Complete
Gluten-Free
Diet & Nutrition Guide

Complete
Gluten-Free
Diet & Nutrition Guide

With a 30-Day Meal Plan & Over 100 Recipes

written by **Alexandra Anca**, MHSc, RD
with **Theresa Santandrea-Cull**

Preface by Dr. Ralph E. Warren, MD, FRCPC, DTM&H

Robert
ROSE

For complete cataloguing information, see page 262.

Disclaimer
This book is a general guide only and should never be a substitute for the skill, knowledge, and experience of a qualified medical professional dealing with the facts, circumstances, and symptoms of a particular case.

The nutritional, medical, and health information presented in this book is based on the research, training, and professional experience of the author, and is true and complete to the best of her knowledge. However, this book is intended only as an informative guide for those wishing to know more about health, nutrition, and medicine; it is not intended to replace or countermand the advice given by the reader's personal physician. Because each person and situation is unique, the author and the publisher urge the reader to check with a qualified health-care professional before using any procedure where there is a question as to its appropriateness. A physician should be consulted before beginning any exercise program. The author and the publisher are not responsible for any adverse effects or consequences resulting from the use of the information in this book. It is the responsibility of the reader to consult a physician or other qualified health-care professional regarding his or her personal care.

This book contains references to products that may not be available everywhere. The intent of the information provided is to be helpful; however, there is no guarantee of results associated with the information provided. Use of brand names is for educational purposes only and does not imply endorsement.

The recipes in this book have been carefully tested by our kitchen and our tasters. To the best of our knowledge, they are safe and nutritious for ordinary use and users. For those people with food or other allergies, or who have special food requirements or health issues, please read the suggested contents of each recipe carefully and determine whether or not they may create a problem for you. All recipes are used at the risk of the consumer.

We cannot be responsible for any hazards, loss, or damage that may occur as a result of any recipe use. For those with special needs, allergies, requirements or health problems, in the event of any doubt, please contact your medical adviser prior to the use of any recipe.

Design and Production: Daniella Zanchetta/PageWave Graphics Inc.
Editors: Bob Hilderley, Senior Editor, Health; Jennifer MacKenzie and Sue Sumeraj, Recipes
Copy editor and indexer: Gillian Watts
Proofreader: Sheila Wawanash
Illustrations: Kveta/Three in a Box
Cover photograph: Colin Erricson

We acknowledge the financial support of the Government of Canada through the Book Publishing Industry Development Program (BPIDP) for our publishing activities.

Published by Robert Rose Inc.
120 Eglinton Avenue East, Suite 800, Toronto, Ontario, Canada M4P 1E2
Tel: (416) 322-6552 Fax: (416) 322-6936
www.robertrose.ca

Printed and bound in Canada
1 2 3 4 5 6 7 8 9 SP 18 17 16 15 14 13 12 11 10

Contents

Preface

> Celiac disease is a unique condition, with a simple therapy — a gluten-free diet for life.

Increasing numbers of North Americans are showing keen interest in the role of nutrition in their health and well-being. It is now unusual to meet an adult who has not been "on a diet" — and many of those who haven't really should be on one. Obesity has become our primary nutritional problem, with a 48% increase in rate over the past 15 years; 66% of American adults and 20% of American children are now overweight. Cardiovascular disease, diabetes, joint problems, and sleep apnea are some of the consequences. The media constantly proclaim the significance of physical fitness, vegetarianism, red meat, trans fats, salt, organic foods, diet clubs, yo-yo diets, and bariatric surgery. It becomes easy to forget that an estimated two-thirds of the world's population, most of them children, fail to receive the minimal daily caloric, protein, and vitamin requirements.

Celiac disease is a common nutritional disorder that has likewise grown in incidence. The prevalence of celiac disease in North America is about 1%, representing, for uncertain reasons, a 4.5 times increase in the past 50 years. Most cases are now diagnosed between the ages of 40 and 60 years, but the disease can be found at any age, including in childhood and among the elderly. The presenting signs and symptoms of celiac disease are both highly variable and sufficiently subtle that the diagnosis is often not reached for 10 years or more. This inordinate delay is often the result of the medical profession's failing to consider or recognize the possibility of celiac disease.

Celiac disease is a unique condition, with a simple therapy — a gluten-free diet for life. This simply stated therapy is not, however, so easy to undertake. The diet is stringent, with challenges that are often overwhelming, yet it is mandatory for recovery, for reversal of established damage if possible, and for maintaining future health. Some celiac patients find it difficult to adapt to this permanently inflexible dietary regime. It doesn't help that the public remains largely ignorant of the disease, including uncertain chefs, indifferent waiters, and unpredictable food companies surreptitiously adding gluten-containing ingredients.

There is light ahead, however. This new millennium has brought us steadily increasing advances in understanding and managing celiac disease. As an autoimmune disease, celiac disease is a genetically predisposed disorder. Patients have a gluten-induced dysfunctional immune system that is both tissue damaging and destructive. We can now unravel complex celiac genetic factors and grasp how they interact with the immune system and gluten metabolism. Sensitive but non-diagnostic screening blood tests are available, and diagnostic small bowel biopsies are more refined. Companies producing gluten-free foods and restaurants offering gluten-free menus have multiplied. Enthusiastic celiac organizations are serving as educational and awareness agencies and support groups. Federal government agencies are promoting appropriate labeling practices and transparency in the selection of food products wherever sold.

Novel and alternative therapies are certain to come in the future, the outcome of painstaking research by medical scientists. Orally administered blockers, inhibitors, antagonists, enzymes, and even a vaccine are being studied. A few clinical trials are already underway, but currently we cannot conclude that these novel therapies will completely replace a gluten-free diet for life.

In this climate, there is an increasing need for dietitians, such as Alexandra Anca, who have special expertise in celiac disease. It is no longer sufficient for newly diagnosed celiac patients to be handed a sheet with two columns listing "Foods Allowed" and "Foods Not Allowed." Once the diagnosis of celiac disease has been confirmed by small bowel biopsies, the celiac dietitian assumes a more important role than the physician in assuring the patient's education, reassurance, and compliance with the gluten-free diet.

Most celiac patients eventually want more in-depth information, not only about gluten-free foods but also about celiac disease itself. This book serves both purposes admirably and provides recipes for preparing nutritious and delicious meals from gluten-free foods. Celiac patients will find joining a celiac organization a good way to keep abreast of new developments, but the popular *Pocket Dictionary: Acceptability of Foods and Food Ingredients for the Gluten-Free Diet* and now the *Complete Gluten-Free Diet & Nutrition Guide* will offer authoritative information and advice.

> The celiac dietitian assumes a more important role than the physician in assuring the patient's education, reassurance, and compliance with the gluten-free diet.

Ralph E. Warren, MD, FRCPC, DTM&H
Member, Professional Advisory Board, Canadian
    Celiac Association
Consultant in Gastroenterology, St. Michael's Hospital
    and the Toronto GI Clinic
Associate Professor of Medicine (ret'd.), University of Toronto

Acknowledgments

We are thankful to Robert Rose Inc. for giving us the opportunity to create this guide. Special thanks to Bob Dees, Bob Hilderley, Sue Sumeraj, Jennifer MacKenzie, Marian Jarkovich, Martine Quibell and all the staff at Robert Rose for their expertise, attention to detail and commitment to excellence. Many thanks to Dr. Ralph Warren and Mavis Molloy, MAEd., RD, for reviewing parts of the book.

From Alexandra:
This book would not have been possible without the influence of my mentors, Dr. Ralph Warren and dietitians Shelley Case, Marion Zarkadas and Mavis Molloy. I am also indebted to the other members of the Professional Advisory Board: Dr. Connie Switzer, Dr. Decker Butzner, Dr. Mohsin Rashid and Vernon Burrows, as well as the members of the executive of the Canadian Celiac Association for their continued support throughout the years.

To those I call my own — Craig and Brooke — thank you for your infinite patience and for giving me the space to focus on this project. Thanks to my parents for their unyielding support and for the opportunity of a new life. To my parents-in-law, thank you for being there for me.

Heartfelt thanks to the physicians and gastroenterologists who supported and cheered me on throughout this project. I am grateful to my patients for the privilege of being part of their lives and their care, and for sharing their stories, challenges and triumphs. I hope this book will make their transition to the gluten-free diet a little easier.

From Theresa:
Many thanks go to Alex, my writing partner in this book adventure. Thank you for choosing me and my recipes. I loved every moment of working with you.

The best job in the world is being a mom, especially Eli and Joseph's mom; thank you guys for choosing me for this honored role. And to my husband, Andrew: without you, there wouldn't be an "us," our family. I love you and us.

Last but not least, to my mom, dad, sisters and brothers, who taught me the meaning of love, life, laughter and family at each and every meal. Thank you. I am very grateful for all of my many blessings.

Introduction

Food stands at the very core of our well-being. It provides us with much-needed energy, comforts us, and connects us with friends and family around the table. No wonder that when food allergies, intolerances, or sensitivities affect us, we become anxious. All of a sudden food becomes our enemy, endangering our health and robbing us of the pleasures of the table. This is the plight of people with celiac disease. Fortunately, a gluten-free diet can restore good health and bring joy back to eating.

Almost a decade ago, I was working in a clinic in midtown Toronto with a team of gastroenterologists, including Dr. Ralph Warren, Associate Professor of Medicine at the University of Toronto and Consultant in Gastroenterology at St. Michael's Hospital. Dr. Warren had been involved with the Canadian Celiac Association for many years as a member of the Professional Advisory Board and as a medical adviser to the Toronto chapter. At the time, celiac disease was not well known among dietitians, but Dr. Warren was keen to educate me. He referred me to a little-known book called the *Pocket Dictionary*, a diet guide for patients newly diagnosed with celiac disease looking to decipher hard-to-read ingredients on food labels so as to avoid gluten in their diet.

However, the dictionary was in dire need of updating. I jumped at the opportunity! It was a huge job that would see me spend more than 1,200 hours in research and involve other dietitians and doctors in the review process. Not surprisingly, I decided to dedicate my practice to the study of celiac disease and development of the gluten-free diet, helping people recognize that this apparently restrictive diet allows them to experiment with foods from various cultures. I couldn't think of a better profession to help those who have to manage the disease. Think about it: there is no medication for celiac disease, only the gluten-free diet. If a dietitian cannot help, who can?

> I jumped at the opportunity! It was a huge job that would see me spend more than 1,200 hours in research and involve other dietitians and doctors in the review process.

As I started counseling more patients suffering from the disease, I listened to their stories of frustration at the outset. Then, little by little, their stories showed signs of hope as they found gluten-free foods they enjoyed and began to share their experiences with friends and family. I also started incorporating gluten-free foods in my own diet and finally got to appreciate quinoa (*keen-wha*), sorghum, amaranth, and many other gluten-free alternatives. I began preparing gluten-free recipes, testing them on my own family. My 3-year-old toddler loves polenta, gluten-free hot cereal in the morning, and amaranth puffs, and when I make quinoa pesto pilaf for dinner, she says, "You make good 'couscous,' Mommy!" (You will find this recipe on page 238).

> Every day, I try to put myself in the shoes of someone with celiac disease as I shop for food and go about my life eating in cafés and restaurants.

Every day, I try to put myself in the shoes of someone with celiac disease as I shop for food and go about my life eating in cafés and restaurants. I have a tremendous respect for patients dealing with this disease. The gluten-free diet is one of the most challenging diets to adopt and comply with. It takes a tremendous amount of hard work, dedication, patience, and diligence to learn the diet and stick to it. But the effort is worth it. After years of suffering miserable symptoms and medical misdiagnoses, individuals who follow a gluten-free diet suddenly feel better. Reconnecting with food becomes their goal, and their most frequent question is, "Now that I know I have celiac disease, what *can* I eat?" Read on for the answer!

Part 1

Celiac Disease Basics

What Is Celiac Disease?

Celiac disease is a genetically based autoimmune condition in which the body attacks itself as a form of self-defense. This chronic immunologic response is triggered by gluten — a portion of the protein present in grains, including wheat, barley, rye, and spelt. This list extends to other grains that are ancient relatives of wheat, such as Kamut, triticale, emmer, and einkorn. The immunologic response to gluten can result in malabsorption of nutrients, leading to a variety of serious health complications.

The intolerance to gluten is permanent and cannot be outgrown even if diagnosed in early childhood. Once considered a rare childhood disease that would eventually be outgrown, celiac disease now affects mostly adults. A very recent study from the Mayo Clinic confirmed that the prevalence of celiac disease has increased more than fourfold in the past 50 years. Globally, epidemiologists estimate that celiac disease may affect 0.5% to 1% of the population, although many cases remain undiagnosed. The only truly effective treatment is adopting a gluten-free diet and restoring nutrient deficiencies with a balanced diet and nutritional supplements.

Genetically based autoimmune conditions

Our immune system provides us with an army of antibodies to fight off antigens (viruses, bacteria, and toxins) that we come into contact with in the air, our food, and our water. The body's first line of defense is the lining of the intestinal tract, which is equipped with white blood cells that produce antibodies called IgA (immunoglobulin A) specific to the gastrointestinal tract's immune system.

When gluten comes into contact with the intestinal lining, the immune system revs up, causing the release of different types of IgA antibodies that instigate an inflammatory process. This process leads to deterioration of the intestinal villi.

Gluten protein fraction

Gluten is a component of the protein found in the endosperm portion of the wheat kernel. Its large size makes it hard to digest. It passes through the stomach, withstands the strength of the churning action, the powerful stomach acid, and protein-digesting enzymes to make its way intact into the duodenum, where it is perceived as toxic by the body's immune system. It is unclear how gluten gets into the mucosal wall, but it may be related to breaks in the mucosal barrier caused by an inflammation involving what is referred to as a leaky gut.

Small Intestine Lining Under Attack

Stomach

Small intestine

Gluten proteins permeate the intestine wall and damage villi

Submucosa

Mucosa

Villi

Lumen

Gluten proteins break through mucosa into the villi

T-cells produce cytokines

B-cells release antibodies

Antigen-presenting cells

Damaged villi

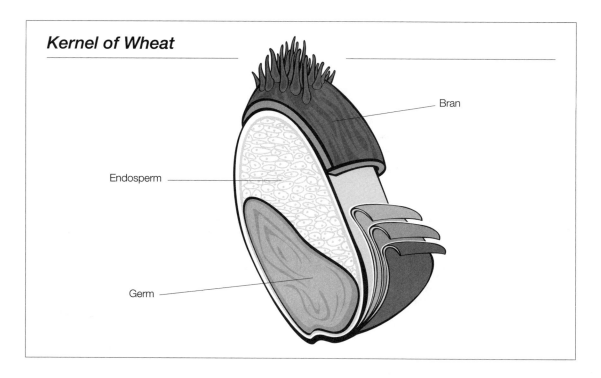

Kernel of Wheat

Bran

Endosperm

Germ

Parts of a kernel

The kernel is the seed from which the plant grows. Each tiny seed contains three distinct parts that are separated during the milling process to produce flour.

> **Endosperm:** makes up about 83% of the kernel weight. It is the source of white endosperm flour. The endosperm contains the greatest share of protein, carbohydrates, and iron, as well as B vitamins such as riboflavin and niacin. It is also a source of soluble fiber.

> **Bran:** makes up about 14% of the kernel weight. The bran contains a small amount of protein, trace minerals, and mostly insoluble dietary fiber.

> **Germ:** makes up about 2.5% of the kernel weight. The germ is the embryo or sprouting section of the seed and contains minimal quantities of high-quality protein and a greater share of B-complex vitamins and trace minerals.

Incidence of celiac disease

Until recently, celiac disease was characteristic of Europe and other developed countries, including the United States, Canada, and Australia. In these countries, it is estimated that 1 in 133 people is diagnosed with celiac disease. New epidemiological studies have shown that the disease is also prevalent in other parts of the world, including the Asian continent and particularly in northern India, where the prevalence of the genes associated with celiac disease in the general population is reported to be 15.6%. Not surprisingly, wheat consumption is higher in the northwestern parts of the country, where cereal is a staple in the diet.

While no specific data are available, high prevalence of celiac disease has also been found in Iran in both the general population and at-risk groups. A high incidence of celiac disease has been reported as well among northern African regions, including Egypt. Interestingly, the highest known incidence of celiac disease occurs in children of the Saharawi tribe of the sub-Saharan desert — 6 out of every 100 children are affected by the disease! In the United States, Canada, and Europe, we know that 1 in 100 children is diagnosed with the disease.

Where Does Celiac Disease Occur?

Celiac disease develops in the gastrointestinal tract (GI tract), or gut. The GI tract is a long, muscular tube that helps food make its way from the mouth, through the esophagus, stomach, small intestine, and large intestine, to the rectum and the anus. It is the site of allergic reactions to foods and autoimmune responses, such as celiac disease. Celiac disease affects the small intestine.

Anatomy of the Digestive Tract

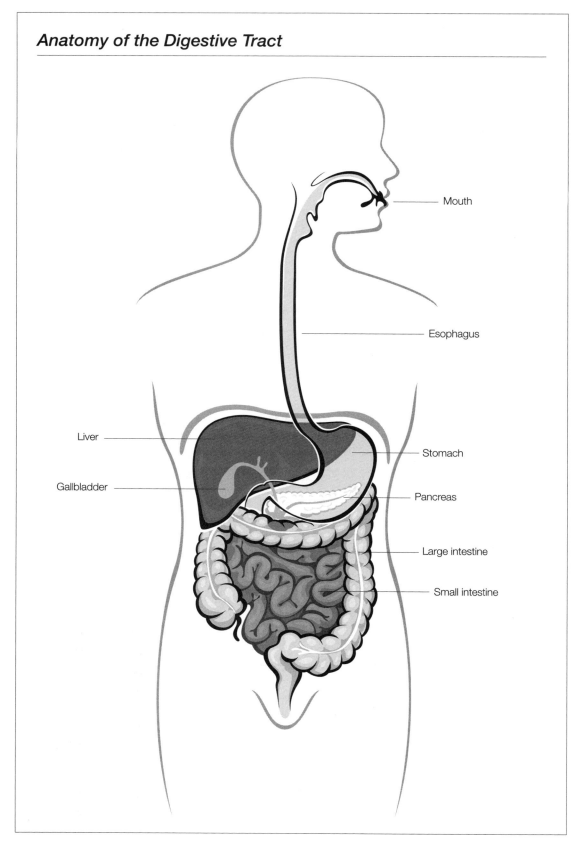

Mouth

Esophagus

Liver

Stomach

Gallbladder

Pancreas

Large intestine

Small intestine

Functions of the GI tract

The primary functions of the gastrointestinal tract are absorption of nutrients and protection against disease. As food is digested in the GI tract, our body extracts the nutrients we need to survive and thrive. Food is broken into small units, which are absorbed into the bloodstream. These nutrients include three macronutrients — carbohydrates, proteins, and fats — as well as various micronutrients — vitamins and minerals. These basic units are essential for fueling our bodies and supporting the function of the main organs.

However, not everything we ingest is food to be digested. Viruses, bacteria, parasites, and other environmental elements that can cause disease also enter our bodies through the GI tract. The entire GI tract, especially the small intestine, manufactures and maintains a strong arsenal of defenses to provide immunity against foreign invaders.

Anatomy of the digestive tract

Celiac disease originates in the GI tract and has an immediate effect on its anatomical components and an associated effect on other body systems, including the neurological, dermatological, and musculoskeletal systems.

Hand to mouth

Digestion starts in the mouth. As you chew, your teeth break large pieces of food into smaller ones, and fluids and saliva blend with those pieces to make them easier to swallow. Your saliva contains starch-digesting enzymes that help kick-start the process of breaking down food into its basic building blocks. After a mouthful of food has been swallowed, it is called a bolus.

Esophagus to stomach

Next, the bolus slides down the esophagus and past the diaphragm into the stomach. The gastroesophageal sphincter closes behind it so that food does not slip back into the esophagus. The stomach cells produce acid secretions that break down food particles. The stomach retains the bolus for a while, adds juices to it, and grinds it into a suspension called chyme. Then, bit by bit, the stomach releases the chyme through the pyloric sphincter into the small intestine, and the pyloric sphincter closes behind it.

Small intestine

At the top of the small intestine, the chyme encounters two fluids dripping into the small intestine from organs attached to the GI tract: the pancreas, the gallbladder, and the liver. The chyme travels down the small intestine through its three segments — the duodenum, the jejunum, and the ileum.

> **Did You Know?**
> **Intestine length**
>
> In the average adult, the small intestine measures about 20 feet (6 meters) in length. The large intestine is wider in diameter than the small intestine, but it measures only 5 feet (1.5 meters) long.

The Small Intestine

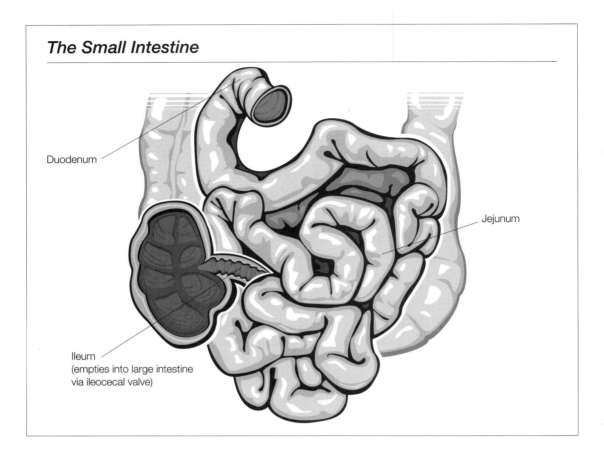

Duodenum

Jejunum

Ileum
(empties into large intestine
via ileocecal valve)

Different parts of the small intestine are more efficient at absorbing different types of nutrients. For example, the duodenum and jejunum are major sites for the absorption of protein, simple sugars, products of fat digestion, iron, calcium, zinc, folate, and the fat-soluble vitamins (K, A, D, and E). A chronic deficiency in iron, calcium, folate, or any of the fat-soluble vitamins can indicate malabsorption caused by a disease or an infection. The ileum is the site of vitamin B_{12} absorption, but when the ileum is damaged by diseases, such as celiac disease or Crohn's disease, vitamin B_{12} deficiency develops.

Large intestine

Having traveled through the segments of the small intestine, the remaining chyme arrives at another sphincter, called the ileocecal valve, at the beginning of the colon (large intestine), in the lower right-hand side of the abdomen. Assuming the digestive tract is healthy, most nutrients are absorbed by the time the chyme reaches the end of the small intestine. What remains consists of water, a few dissolved salts, some bodily secretions (mucus), and fiber. In the colon, healthy bacteria degrade some of the fiber even further, while fluid (water) and electrolytes (sodium and potassium) are reabsorbed back into the body.

When it comes to absorption, the small intestine is actually one of the most elegantly designed organ systems in the body. In its 20 feet (6 meters), it provides a surface comparable to a quarter of a football field in area that engulfs and absorbs the nutrient molecules. While the inner surface of the intestine looks smooth and slippery, when viewed under the microscope it turns out to be wrinkled into hundreds of folds. Each fold, in turn, is covered with thousands of small projections called villi. A single villus, magnified even more, turns out to be composed of hundreds of cells, each covered with microscopic hairs called microvilli. The villi are in constant motion, wiggling and squirming much like the tentacles found on marine corals. Any nutrient molecule small enough to be absorbed is trapped within the microvilli and passed directly into the bloodstream. Others that are only partially digested are also caught in the microvilli, digested by enzymes there, and absorbed into the cells.

Rectum and anus

The remaining waste matter is excreted periodically into the rectum and then through the anus.

What Causes Celiac Disease?

Individuals with celiac disease have the genetic makeup to develop it, but this potential is triggered by environmental and immunologic factors.

Genetic factors

This disease is inherited; it runs in the family. A first-degree sibling has a 40% chance of also inheriting the disease. In the general population, there is a 7% to 20% chance that any member of the family of an individual affected with celiac disease may also carry the same genetic makeup.

Who should be screened for celiac disease?

- **Children:** In children, detecting celiac disease is imperative to ensure that nutrients are absorbed optimally while they are still growing and to prevent future complications. It may also be necessary to screen children more than once, since celiac disease may be silent during childhood.
- **First-degree relatives:** Parents, brothers and sisters should also be tested, particularly if they suffer from gastrointestinal symptoms or simply have other long-standing conditions that have not improved.

The two specific genes that have been recognized so far in celiac disease are part of the HLA class. The proteins found on white blood cells that are encoded by genes HLA-DQ2 and HLA-DQ8 are primed to interact with gluten. About 95% of individuals with celiac disease have the HLA-DQ2 gene, while only 5% have the HLA-DQ8.

Lately, however, it has become clear that the genetic makeup of celiac disease is not limited to these two types of genes. In fact, to date, at least 13 additional candidate genes have been identified as contributing to celiac disease.

Screening

More than 50% of patients with celiac disease have a family member with undiagnosed disease. Children, siblings, and parents of people diagnosed with celiac disease should be tested because they carry a high risk of being carriers of DQ2 and DQ8. Screening for celiac disease includes blood tests and a small intestine tissue biopsy. Genetic testing may be useful in some cases.

Environmental factors

The environmental trigger in the genetically susceptible person is gluten, the protein fraction found in wheat, barley, rye, spelt, and Kamut. These proteins are called gliadins in wheat, hordeins in barley, and secalins in rye. In the past, the avenin protein in oats was also included in the list.

However, oats are known to be more closely related to rice and a more distant genetic relative of wheat, barley, and rye. Currently there is concern over cross-contamination of commercially available oats with gluten-containing grains during harvesting, transportation, and milling.

Did You Know?
Oats consensus

There is an increased consensus that pure, uncontaminated oats are safe when consumed in moderate amounts. This position has been adopted by a number of celiac organizations, research centers, and government associations. Nevertheless, some organizations continue to recommend restricting the use of oats in newly diagnosed patients, while others, such as the Coeliac Society of Australia, recommend complete avoidance of even pure, uncontaminated oats.

Immunologic factors

In a person with an HLA-DQ2 or HLA-DQ8 genetic makeup who is exposed to gluten in the environment, there need only be a switch, such as a gastrointestinal infection, pregnancy, or surgical procedure, to turn on the immunologic response that produces the symptoms of celiac disease.

Antibodies and antigens

When gluten comes into contact with the intestinal lining, the immune system revs up, causing the release of different types of IgA antibodies that instigate an inflammatory process. This process leads to deterioration of the intestinal villi. Because these antibodies are specific for their interaction with gluten, blood tests measuring their concentration in the bloodstream are very accurate.

What Are the Symptoms of Celiac Disease?

Celiac disease can surface in many different ways. Almost every system of your body may be affected. This very wide spectrum of symptoms is also a reason why celiac disease can take a long time to diagnose. Not only do symptoms range in severity but they affect everyone differently. Some individuals become violently ill the minute they ingest a piece of bread or a bite of a wheat cracker. Others may have long-standing iron deficiency anemia that they keep treating with iron supplements without any resolution. Celiac disease can range from severe to mild in its symptoms. Those who are very symptomatic will seek ongoing medical care. Those with very few symptoms may find the diagnosis an annoyance.

Gluten sensitivity versus celiac disease

While in celiac *disease* gluten triggers an autoimmune reaction causing damage to the intestinal lining, in gluten *sensitivity* it causes only abdominal symptoms. Individuals with gluten sensitivity will experience bloating, constipation, and cramping, but there will be no underlying damage to the intestines, nor will they suffer from any complications such as nutrient deficiencies or metabolic, hormonal, and neurological disorders. For these people, simply taking gluten out of the diet will make them feel better.

Symptoms of celiac disease

Gastrointestinal
- Chronic diarrhea or constipation
- Flatulence, bloating, abdominal pain
- Nausea and vomiting, especially in children
- Gastroesophageal reflux

Skin
- Severe itching rash (dermatitis herpetiformis)
- Easy bruising

Physiological and metabolic
- Anemias and deficiencies in iron, folic acid, and vitamin B_{12}
- Deficiencies in vitamins A, D, E, and K
- Lactose intolerance
- Abnormalities in liver blood tests (e.g., liver enzymes)
- Extreme weakness and fatigue
- Weight loss (although individuals may be overweight or of normal weight when first diagnosed)

Oral
- Mouth ulcers
- Defects in dental enamel

Musculoskeletal system
- Bone and joint pain
- Swelling of hands and ankles
- Short stature (although the presence of normal or tall stature does not exclude celiac disease)

Reproductive system
- Amenorrhea
- Infertility (men and women)
- Recurrent miscarriages

Neurological system
- Headaches, including migraines
- Depression
- Mood swings
- Tingling, predominantly in the hands and feet (peripheral neuropathy)
- Gait disturbance (gluten ataxia)
- Epilepsy (with or without cerebral calcifications)

In very young children, symptoms may include
- Diarrhea
- Nausea and vomiting
- Abdominal distention
- Failure to thrive

Older children and teenagers may experience
- Short stature
- Severe irritability
- Delayed puberty
- Dental enamel defects

Atypical celiac disease

Sometimes celiac disease may affect only the proximal (or uppermost) part of the small intestine instead of reaching far down and causing many of the classical gastrointestinal symptoms. In this case, affected individuals develop only single nutrient deficiencies, such as iron or calcium deficiency, that can lead to various conditions, such as osteopenia, osteoporosis, and anemia. Some of these patients may also have mild gastrointestinal symptoms, such as bloating, constipation, and indigestion, which usually get diagnosed as irritable bowel syndrome.

Associated conditions

Although celiac disease tends to occur on its own, it is associated with a number of other conditions. If you are suffering from any of the following conditions, you are at a higher risk of having celiac disease and should consider being tested:

- Diabetes (type 1 insulin-dependent diabetes mellitus)
- Thyroid disease
- Osteoporosis
- Autoimmune liver disease
- Down syndrome
- Turner syndrome
- Selective IgA deficiency
- Sjögren's syndrome (dry-mouth syndrome)
- Cardiomyopathy
- Addison's disease
- T-cell lymphoma

Malabsorption symptoms

If celiac disease spreads downward in the small intestine, absorption of fat-soluble vitamins, such as A, D, E, and K, is affected.

- **Vitamin A deficiency:** visual and reproductive problems
- **Vitamin D deficiency:** rickets (in children), osteopenia, and osteoporosis
- **Vitamin E deficiency:** neurological symptoms, such as "pins and needles" sensations in hands and feet or unsteadiness of gait
- **Vitamin K deficiency:** easy bruising and bleeding

Nutrient deficiencies typically develop with undiagnosed celiac disease and can result in serious complications.

- **Iron deficiency:** anemia, fatigue, weakness
- **Calcium deficiency:** osteopenia, osteoporosis
- **Folate deficiency:** anemia, fatigue, weakness
- **Vitamin B_{12} deficiency:** in severe cases, may lead to fatigue and weakness

Did You Know?
Weight factor

Classic images of thin, wasted, and severely malnourished individuals with celiac disease seen in textbooks are rarely seen in clinical practice. Being at normal weight or overweight does not rule out celiac disease.

Did You Know?
Secondary lactose intolerance

This condition develops as celiac disease worsens, damaging or destroying the source of the lactase enzymes in the small bowel's mucosal lining. Bloating, gas, and diarrhea result from ingestion of milk and milk products.

Erin is a 24-year-old recent university graduate. She came to the consultation accompanied by her mother. Her story began when she was about 4 or 5 and started experiencing strong reactions to different foods, including pasta, bread, and cookies. The reactions were mostly bloating, gas, and pain. It felt as if anything she ate would make her sick, so she avoided most foods. For most of the time she was irritable and was told to stop acting up. She developed anemia and became lactose intolerant. Her growth was stunted in her early teenage years, and she felt rundown and tired most of the time. Her family physician sent her to numerous allergy specialists in a quest to pinpoint specific food allergies, but those tests were inconclusive. She continued to experience anemia and feelings of lethargy through most of her high school years and into university. She blamed that on her workload — despite her ill health, she was pushing herself to complete school and hold down a part-time job to pay for undergraduate studies.

Just as she was entering university, she decided to consult a naturopathic doctor, who suggested that she avoid all wheat and dairy products. She started the diet, avoiding the most obvious sources of wheat — bread, pasta, couscous, breaded and baked foods — and choosing lactose-free foods, and immediately felt better. However, about 6 months into the diet, she noticed that the symptoms had returned and were more intense than ever. Her blood iron levels continued to be low, and painful gas and bloating became even more bothersome.

That's when she decided to seek a second opinion from another physician, who suggested she investigate celiac disease as a possible diagnosis. Not surprisingly, her blood test for IgA-tTG antibodies was well above normal. She was referred to a gastroenterologist to confirm the diagnosis with a small bowel biopsy. The biopsy was positive for celiac disease and confirmed that she had been on a gluten-free diet because the intestinal lining had started to heal somewhat. Erin was lucky: had she been more diligent about implementing a gluten-free diet prior to being tested for celiac disease, the biopsy would have given a false negative result and her diagnosis would have continued to be uncertain. She was also sent for a bone density scan because osteoporosis is a complication of undiagnosed celiac disease.

How Is Celiac Disease Diagnosed?

Many people with celiac disease tell stories about years spent seeing doctors, specialists, and other health-care professionals in search of an answer to their symptoms. Others counter with tales of experiencing a gut feeling — no pun intended — that they had celiac disease and insisting on being tested. There are several ways to test for celiac disease. The most important is a small intestine biopsy, which is the gold standard for diagnosis. There are other, less invasive tests you may want to try before undergoing a biopsy.

Malabsorption tests

Several non-invasive tests for malabsorption can be used to decide if a biopsy should be performed. These markers are measured by blood tests only:

- Hemoglobin
- Iron
- Folate
- Vitamin B$_{12}$
- Vitamin D

Endoscopy

To take a biopsy of the small intestine, a gastroenterologist will perform an endoscopy, using intravenous sedation. A scope is inserted through the mouth down toward the duodenum. Since the pattern of villi atrophy from celiac disease may be patchy, the gastroenterologist will take multiple samples to increase the likelihood of detecting areas that have been damaged by the disease. These biopsies are then sent to a pathologist, who will be looking for variable degrees of damage compatible with celiac disease.

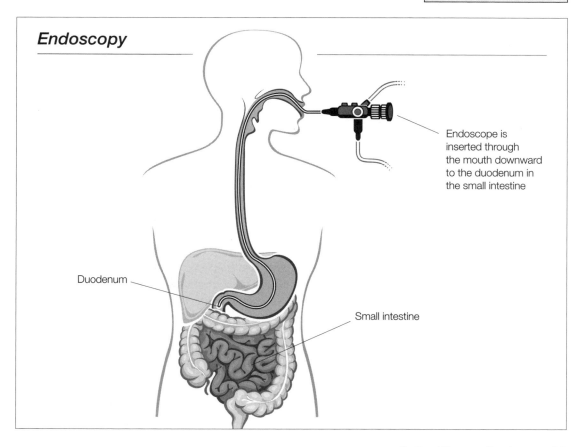

Endoscopy

Endoscope is inserted through the mouth downward to the duodenum in the small intestine

Duodenum

Small intestine

Blood tests

Currently there are two serological (blood) tests commonly used in clinical practice to screen for celiac disease: IgA endomysial antibody (EMA) and IgA tissue transglutaminase antibody (tTG). Serum IgA antibody levels must be obtained to exclude false negative results, since 1 in 40 celiacs is serum IgA deficient, compared to 1 in 400 for the normal population.

EMA test

The IgA endomysial antibody (EMA) is highly specific for celiac disease and has a high correlation to the degree of villous atrophy. This means that if the test is positive and the individual is not deficient in IgA antibodies, celiac disease is likely to be present. However, if the person is IgA deficient, this test will falsely indicate absence of celiac disease. Another instance that may present with false negative IgA EMA blood tests is in children under 2, where this type of antibody is not present.

Reliability of blood tests

Serological tests have come a long way. One of the latest tests, available at some pharmacies in Canada and parts of Europe, allows individuals to qualitatively screen for elevated levels of IgA-tTG antibody in the comfort of their own home. Despite how simple it sounds, the test needs to be properly administered and is insufficient for detection and proper diagnosis of celiac disease. If the result is positive, it should be followed up by a standard tTG antibody test performed on a sample of venous blood, and then referral to a gastroenterologist for biopsies. The test is a convenient tool for screening those with minimal symptoms and individuals who are at low risk of celiac disease.

Another recently available test, the IgA deaminated gliadin peptide antibody test (IgA-DGP), has a similar accuracy to the IgA-tTG test and may be considered as an additional screening tool.

The reality is that none of the serological tests are 100% specific or sensitive for celiac disease. The single most definitive test remains the small intestine biopsy.

---

tTG

IgA tissue transglutaminase (tTG) is an enzyme that binds to gluten and turns it into a toxic molecule. This coupling triggers the autoimmune response characteristic of celiac disease. The combination is recognized by the body's immune system as an antigen. Therefore, the presence of abnormally high levels of IgA-tTG in the blood may indicate the presence of celiac disease. However, the tTG antibody may also be abnormally high in the presence of other conditions, such as diabetes, liver disease, and even Crohn's disease. Nevertheless, the IgA-tTG antibody test is still a highly specific and fairly sensitive marker for celiac disease.

Gluten challenge

If individuals have started a gluten-free diet prior to diagnosis, all screening blood tests may show normal results and a proper diagnosis could easily be missed. If the gastroenterologist suspects celiac disease, a gluten challenge may be recommended. This involves consuming gluten-containing foods daily for 3 months or more, depending on your symptoms.

However, there are no clear recommendations on how to perform this challenge or what markers to rely on for timing the biopsy after the challenge. Some specialists recommend that the amount of gluten ingested be equivalent to 4 slices of bread per day for a minimum of 3 months. If patients can tolerate this amount without major symptoms, a 3-month period or longer is preferred in order to ensure accurate diagnosis. Considering that a slice of bread is estimated to contain up to 3.5 grams of gluten, the suggested standard would mean ingesting approximately 14 grams of gluten every day for the recommended length of time.

Remember that celiac disease affects individuals differently and the damage to the intestinal lining is not uniform. This means that some individuals may need to consume less than this amount for histopathology to change, while others may need to administer the gluten challenge for even longer than 3 months.

However, in a recent study, researchers have shown through a double-blind, placebo-controlled prospective study design (which included quantitative measures of small intestinal biopsies) that 50 mg of daily gluten ingestion for 3 months was sufficient to cause significant changes in the small bowel mucosa of treated celiac patients.

CASE HISTORY
Challenging the gluten challenge

Michelle visited our clinic complaining of her 3-year-old son. Since birth he had been very slow to grow and put on weight. When he turned 2, he started developing diarrhea, puffy eyes, and a swollen belly. He became cranky and irritable. His pediatrician suspected possible celiac disease and advised Michelle to start her son on a gluten-free diet. "Within a short period of time," Michelle explained, "my son improved so much I couldn't recognize him! It's as if I had found another person! He was so much calmer, happier; his belly was no longer distended; his bowels were normal. He finally ate what I cooked for him!" But Michelle still wanted to find out what the diagnosis was. Was it celiac disease? Was it gluten sensitivity? Or was it something else?

When I told her about the need to go on a gluten challenge, Michelle immediately objected. "There is no way I can go back to giving him gluten now! I would have to take a month off work, he would be so miserable! What else can I do?"

I suggested genetic testing to rule out celiac disease.

Dermatitis herpetiformis (DH) is frequently misdiagnosed as eczema or another skin condition and treated with topical creams. After initial treatment fails to clear the blisters and itchy rashes, dermatologists will typically order a skin biopsy from an unaffected skin area close to an erupted blister. If the skin biopsy is positive for DH, there is no need for an intestinal biopsy. A positive skin biopsy is a confirmed diagnosis for celiac disease.

Genetic testing

Genetic testing involves detection of the DQ2 or DQ8 alleles that are closely associated with celiac disease. The tests use a blood sample, saliva, or cells obtained by swabbing the inside of the cheek.

Genetic testing may help in one of two ways. First, it can rule out celiac disease in nearly all cases. This means that an individual with a negative gene test does not have the genetic predisposition for celiac disease and is not likely to develop it. People who test negative for the gene would not be required to have regular antibody screening for the remainder of their lives. For example, the children of an adult with celiac disease could have the gene test. The results would allow the parent to know which children needed close monitoring. However, keep in mind that more than a dozen newly discovered genes are also thought to contribute to the development of celiac disease, which would make a negative gene test not 100% definitive.

Genetic testing may also be somewhat useful for individuals who have been on a gluten-free diet for a significant period of time but have not been properly diagnosed with celiac disease through a biopsy. For a person who faces this situation, a negative gene test would indicate that the symptoms are not the result of celiac disease. A positive gene test, however, does not diagnose the disease but does increase the likelihood that it is present.

Only about 30% to 35% of populations where celiac disease is prevalent carry the HLA-DQ2 or HLA-DQ8 genes, with only 2% to 5% of this group actually developing the disease. This means that celiac disease may have other genes associated with it or that other, environmental factors contribute to the development of the disease.

How Will This Disease Affect My Life?

Celiac disease is a lifelong illness that can lead to complications and associated conditions if not properly diagnosed and treated. The primary treatment is to avoid gluten-containing foods and to restore nutrient deficiencies. There is also a psychological factor involved in treating celiac disease because it affects your quality of life. Coming to terms with the disease is not always easy.

Quality of life

At first you may be relieved that after many years of suffering miserable symptoms, someone is able to tell you what is wrong, but as news of the diagnosis sets in, celiac disease can feel like a life sentence.

A study at the Celiac Disease Center at Columbia University found that people with celiac disease had many difficulties maintaining a healthy social and family life while trying to adhere to the gluten-free diet. In this study, 86% of participants reported difficulties when dining out, 82% found it difficult to travel, and 67% said that celiac disease negatively impacted their family life.

Denial

You may not want to talk about the diagnosis and gluten sensitivity. That's a normal feeling. Most of us have to contend with some health condition, but we seldom need to divulge it publicly, unless we do so by choice. Despite our health, we want to remain connected to our group and maintain a sense of belonging. However, when you have celiac disease, inevitable exposure to food forces you to admit it. If you continue not to disclose your gluten sensitivity, it can lead to further feelings of being an outsider.

Resentment

You may start resenting that you can no longer eat what you want and cannot go to restaurants without calling ahead to see if they have gluten-free dishes. Inquiring about gluten-free options may sometimes be met with a reply that only reflects ignorance on the part of restaurant staff: "Oh, you're on a high-protein diet! Sure, we can accommodate you." You want to carry on with your life, enjoy the spontaneity of going out, being social, and yet you must always be on guard. The fear of being contaminated with gluten puts pressure on those with celiac disease, not only at restaurants but also in family situations. When a close family member goes to the trouble of making a special meal for you and they assure you it is gluten-free, you find it hard to refuse or ask numerous questions. You may feel misunderstood, isolated and no longer able to fit in.

Feeling neglected

Other people feel neglected. One woman described the following experience: "I was at a 25th birthday party given by a friend who served pie and salad. I ate a little salad. I was very sad and very disappointed. Excuse me for existing…"

Information overload

Others are simply overwhelmed by the amount of information they have to process about which foods they can and cannot eat. Most people diagnosed with celiac disease spend countless hours on the telephone with food companies trying to find out if products are indeed gluten-free. Sometimes the information is misleading and feelings of mistrust set in.

> **Did You Know?**
> **Unwanted visibility**
>
> Relationships with family members, friends, relatives, and co-workers can become difficult when your food intolerance becomes the main topic of conversation. Some people describe this as a gluten-intolerance fixation, which they find uncomfortable.

Self-control

Then comes a stage of self-control as you find ways to manage the gluten-free diet and lessen its initial negative impact on your emotional and social life. Years into the diagnosis, when much of the information has been digested, many patients report that celiac disease is a blessing in disguise.

Countless patients are upbeat about the gluten-free diet, believing it to be much healthier, and are grateful for not having to rely on processed foods. They feel empowered by adopting a healthier lifestyle and finding a support network that understands their situation. Their food diaries show a high consumption of fruits, vegetables, fresh meat, dairy, and legumes, along with a new appreciation for healthy gluten-free grains. Steering away from processed foods allows them to better appreciate home-cooked meals. In fact, in my years of practice, I have noticed that patients who cook their meals at home find it easiest to adapt to the gluten-free diet.

CASE HISTORY
Suffering in silence

Mildred was recently diagnosed with celiac disease at age 82 and confessed, "I cannot believe it has taken my entire life to be diagnosed. I suffered in silence, but I always suspected a reaction to wheat. It all started after the birth of my first child. I remember having symptoms: terrible cramps, constipation, sore bones, lactose intolerance, and thyroid disease. I saw many doctors for every one of my conditions and had many tests and X-rays, but celiac disease never came up. I was diagnosed through a small bowel biopsy and started the gluten-free diet. It changed my life!"

Who Will Take Care of Me?

Once you begin to accept your diagnosis, it is time to plan your recovery. Every patient diagnosed with celiac disease needs nutritional counseling by a health-care professional with expertise in celiac disease. There will be a need for routine checkups to ensure that the gluten-free diet is working and that healing has begun. Take control of your medical care by assembling your team of health-care professionals and keeping a chart of your progress. Your health is your most important asset, one that deserves your utmost attention.

Celiac disease management team

While you may plan to assemble a full team of professionals to manage your conditions, not all members listed here may be available in your community. Don't worry. Work with the professionals who are available. Many can handle more than one responsibility.

1. Dietitian with expertise in celiac disease to
    - Assess vitamin and mineral deficiencies as well as overall nutritional status
    - Analyze nutritional content of current diet to determine areas of improvement
    - Assess barriers to implementation or answer specific questions about food products or strategies to be used in restaurants, on outings, at social gatherings
    - Design gluten-free and nutrient-rich meal plans and recipes

2. Naturopathic doctor with expertise in celiac disease to
    - Establish nutritional supplement protocols and safe dosages
    - Address quality of life and lifestyle concerns

3. Pharmacist with expertise in clinical nutrition to
    - Check all prescription medication for presence of gluten
    - Check all vitamin and mineral supplements for presence of gluten or ingredients derived from gluten-containing products
    - Check medicinal or non-medicinal ingredients in natural health products

4. Gastroenterologist to
    - Obtain biopsies to confirm diagnosis
    - Check on overall clinical recovery and ensure that patient is doing well (i.e., gaining weight, recovering from iron deficiency, increasing in energy, decreasing in abdominal discomfort, returning to normal bowel functions)
    - Consider repeating biopsy at 2 to 5 years, or earlier, if patient has persistent symptoms despite being on the gluten-free diet

5. Family physician with knowledge of your medical history to
    - Coordinate the team
    - Help interpret information for you
    - Encourage compliance
    - Address family concerns

My Health Chart

To help keep control of your condition and the treatments your team of health-care professionals prescribe, you may want to keep your own medical chart. Update it or augment it as you learn more about your condition. Ask your health-care providers for assistance and carry this chart with you as you visit their offices.

My Name: _____ Date of Birth: _____

Medications

Are you taking any medications? Yes / No
If Yes, what and why? _____
_____
_____

Nutritional supplements

Do you take any vitamin/mineral/herbal supplements? Yes / No
If Yes, what and why? _____
_____
_____

Food sensitivities

Do you have other food sensitivities, intolerances, or allergies? Yes / No
If Yes, what and when did they start? _____
_____
_____
_____

Laboratory tests

Endoscopy biopsy results _____
IgA-tTG _____ IgA _____ IgA-EMA _____
Iron _____
Vitamin B_{12} _____
Folate _____
Bone mineral density _____
Albumin (urine) _____
CBC (blood count) _____

Symptoms

[Use boxes to check off]

[ ] Diarrhea, runny stools
[ ] Bloating
[ ] Stomach cramping
[ ] Joint pain

[ ] Itchy skin
[ ] Easy bruising
[ ] Frequent headache
[ ] Mood swings
[ ] Tingling in hands and feet
[ ] Gait disturbance
[ ] Extreme weakness and fatigue
[ ] Weight loss (although individuals may be overweight or of normal weight when first diagnosed)

Associated Conditions

[Use boxes to check off]

[ ] Diabetes mellitus (type 1)
[ ] Thyroid disease
[ ] Osteoporosis
[ ] Irritable bowel syndrome
[ ] Lactose intolerance
[ ] Dental enamel defects
[ ] T-cell lymphoma
[ ] Other autoimmune disorders:
- Autoimmune liver disease (such as primary biliary cirrhosis)
- Down syndrome (a genetic disorder)
- Turner syndrome (a genetic disorder)
- Selective IgA deficiency
- Sjögren's syndrome (dry-mouth syndrome)
- Cardiomyopathy (inflammatory disorder of the heart muscle)
- Addison's disease (atrophy or shrinking of the adrenal glands)
- Aphthous stomatitis (canker sores)

Pediatrics

Percentile Growth (girls) _____
Percentile Growth (boys) _____

Medical History

What medical conditions have you been treated for in the past? When?

_____
_____
_____

Family History

What medical conditions have your immediate family members been treated for?
Any food sensitivities, allergies, or intolerances? Any celiac disease symptoms?

_____
_____
_____

Diet Diary

Keeping a diet diary or daily record of what you eat and how you feel may help you to manage your condition and give clues to your health-care team about where to look for causes. Here is an example of a 1-day or 24-hour diet diary. You will likely want to keep it for 3 to 7 days to see if any trends emerge.

Tips for getting the most out of your food diary

- Pick 3 typical days (2 weekdays and 1 weekend day) to reflect regular eating habits.
- Record the information as soon as you finish eating so that the quantities, types of foods and brand names are fresh in your memory.
- Don't forget to record what you drank (water, coffee, pop, juice).
- When estimating the amount of food consumed, it's best to stick to familiar measurements (1 cup, 1 tablespoon, 1 teaspoon).
- Record any intake of additional fat from margarine, added oils, salad dressing or mayonnaise. It's best to approximate the quantity you used in teaspoons.
- For home-cooked meals, it would be ideal to record the recipe and estimate the servings you consumed.

Meal/Time	What did I eat?	How much?	My mood and/or symptoms
Breakfast			
Morning snack			

Meal/Time	What did I eat?	How much?	My mood and/ or symptoms
Lunch			
Afternoon snack			
Dinner			
Evening snack			

CASE HISTORY
Good prognosis

Mary is a 57-year-old white woman who had been recently diagnosed with celiac disease when she met with us for the first time. She was overweight but otherwise reasonably healthy and showed early signs of osteopenia. No other symptoms were reported. At her annual physical exam, blood work revealed moderately elevated serum aspartate aminotransferase (AST) and alanine aminotransferase (ALT) activity, markers for liver damage. She enjoyed drinking on rare occasions, having only 1 to 2 glasses of white wine when dining out. There was no history of celiac disease or liver disease or colon cancer in the family, and all other blood work was unremarkable.

Because of her abnormal liver enzyme values, she was sent for further testing, including a referral to a gastroenterologist. Further blood work revealed elevated IgA-tTG with no deficiency of IgA antibodies. She underwent a small bowel biopsy, which confirmed the diagnosis of celiac disease. Soon after, Mary was referred to us for nutrition counseling and placed on a gluten-free diet.

When we asked her how she felt about the diagnosis, she revealed being completely surprised and, frankly, doubted that she had been given the correct diagnosis. She had no history of celiac disease in the family and none of the typical symptoms associated with celiac disease: weight loss, diarrhea, bloating, gas, or constipation. She was most concerned about not being able to identify the times when she might accidentally ingest gluten, since her symptoms were silent. She had been told that the gluten-free diet would reverse the liver damage within a year of good adherence to the diet.

With a bit of hesitation, she went about changing her diet and eating mostly home-cooked meals to increase her control over ingredients and sources of cross-contamination. She started carrying snacks with her and explored gluten-free baking. She found a supportive group of friends who chose to organize potluck lunches instead of eating out. On these occasions Mary would share her own gluten-free meals and try new gluten-free recipes prepared by her friends. While on the gluten-free diet, she noticed that she increased her intake of fruits and vegetables, which helped her weight loss goals.

The suggested gluten-free menu plan we designed for her included strategies for both weight loss and increased calcium intake from foods. Since she was not lactose intolerant, dietary calcium was easily obtained from low-fat dairy products and gluten-free non-dairy products in order to slow down the effects of osteopenia. To her relief, at her 6 month follow-up the AST/ALT values had dropped significantly and were within normal values. All her efforts had been worthwhile! The challenge remained that she would continue to maintain a 100% gluten-free diet, all the while avoiding cross-contamination or accidental gluten ingestion.

Part 2

The Gluten-Free Diet

The Gluten-Free Diet

How to manage celiac disease is no mystery — simply avoid gluten in your diet. If only it were so easy. What foods with gluten content should you avoid? What can you substitute for gluten-containing foods? What foods can you enjoy without risk? These are more complicated questions.

Getting to know how to eat a gluten-free diet is challenging. You need to be patient and persistent. Give yourself the time to experiment with new foods and allow yourself to fail — this is how you learn best. Remember that it took you a long time to be diagnosed and you are now on your way to recovery. Having a positive attitude and a reliable source of information is the key to mastering this new way of eating. It's just like learning a new job — the job of eating properly to manage celiac disease. Along the way, you will discover the strength to make changes in your lifestyle. And the recipes in this book will amaze you at how simple and delicious the gluten-free diet really is!

Gluten Limits

How much gluten can I have? This is the most common question asked by patients who are newly diagnosed with celiac disease. Andrew, 75 years old, newly diagnosed, wanted to know his gluten limits. "I really like my soda bread. Can I have a slice once in a while?" The only treatment for celiac disease is a 100% gluten-free diet. While no health professional would ever deviate from this recommendation, life all around us is not gluten-free, and gluten contamination of other foods is very common.

While sources of hidden gluten are becoming rare as labeling laws require manufacturers to declare sources of allergens on food labels, gluten-free foods may sometimes be contaminated with trace amounts of gluten. Recent studies found that 15% of so-called gluten-free foods in Canada and 30% in Europe had more than 20 parts per million of gluten. In the Canadian study, about half of the contaminated samples were flours such as buckwheat flour and cornmeal, and the rest were cooked processed foods, but the contamination levels were similar.

One of the latest studies shows that as little as 50 mg of gluten a day for 3 months can cause damage to the intestinal lining. Consider that a slice of bread is estimated to contain as much as 3.5 grams of gluten, which amounts to about 70 times this 50 mg threshold for damage. In other words, it takes as little as a bread crumb ($\frac{1}{70}$th of a slice of bread) to inadvertently start the inflammatory process and intestinal damage. Because of the small number of patients in this study, no firm conclusions could be made about the effect of ingesting less than 10 mg of gluten daily. This remains a gray area for research. As a dietitian, I encourage you to give 100% effort to following the gluten-free diet. Because even your best effort may be thwarted by cross-contamination, you need to be vigilant about accidental ingestion of glutenous food.

Gluten-free standards

What is the standard for gluten-free foods? When is a food considered gluten-free? Until recently, the standard was different depending on where you happened to be. This is changing and we are getting closer to an international standard.

The Codex Alimentarius, or food code, is the international reference point for consumers, food producers and processors, national food control agencies, and the international food trade.

Gluten-free definitions

The Codex Standard for Foods for Special Dietary Use for Persons Intolerant to Gluten defines gluten-free foods as those

a. Derived or made with ingredients that do not contain wheat (i.e., all *Triticum* species, such as durum wheat, spelt, and Kamut), rye, barley, oats, or their crossbred varieties, and the gluten level does not exceed 20 parts per million in total, based on the food as sold or distributed to the consumer.
b. Derived or made with ingredients from wheat (i.e., all *Triticum* species, such as durum wheat, spelt, and Kamut), rye, barley, or oats, or their crossbred varieties that have been specially processed to remove gluten, not exceeding 20 parts per million in total, based on the food as sold or distributed to the consumer.

The United States Food and Drug Administration (FDA) is proposing to define the term "gluten-free" for voluntary use in labeling of foods to mean that a food does not contain the following:

a. An ingredient from any species of wheat, barley, or rye, or crossbred varieties of these grains. This list does not include oats. Oat products labeled gluten-free must contain less than 20 parts per million of gluten.

b. An ingredient that is derived from a prohibited grain that has not been processed to remove gluten, such as wheat bran, wheat flour, hydrolyzed wheat protein, malt syrup, or malt extract.
c. An ingredient that is derived from a prohibited grain that has been processed to remove gluten, but the use of the ingredient exceeds 20 parts per million of gluten in the food.
d. 20 parts per million or more of gluten.

Currently in Canada the definition of the term "gluten-free" refers to "a food that does not contain wheat, including spelt and Kamut, or oats, barley, rye or triticale or any part thereof." Canada has not accepted the Codex standard for gluten-free foods; however, Health Canada is currently working on developing a definition for the use of the term "gluten-free."

The European Commission has approved use of the new Codex standard as the basis for a law on labeling of food for people who are gluten intolerant. The law came into effect in January 2009, but manufacturers have until January 2012 to comply with the law, allowing time for manufacturers to comply to product ranges and change product labels.

Created in the 1960s by the World Health Organization (WHO) and the Food and Agriculture Organization of the United Nations (FAO), the Codex Alimentarius Commission — the body charged with developing the food code — has reviewed all important aspects of food pertaining to the protection of consumer health and fair practices in the food trade.

Foods to Avoid

The cornerstone of the gluten-free diet is to avoid a long list of foods. At first glance, this list is quite overwhelming. It seems like everything has wheat, barley, or rye as an ingredient. As Andrea, newly diagnosed with celiac disease, complained, "I didn't know all these foods have gluten! I can't believe how much there is to learn. I feel so guilty when I end up eating gluten by mistake." Don't feel guilty. Just keep on your toes and stay alert. Soon you won't be tricked by food advertisements and well-intended but sometimes misleading advice.

Two tips for avoiding gluten

Here are two simple guidelines to follow when starting your gluten-free diet:

1. Choose fresh, whole foods instead of processed ones. This may not be as convenient as eating processed foods, but the result is often tastier and healthier.
2. Read the food label every time. Food manufacturers change formulations at short notice, and what you thought may be gluten-free today may not be tomorrow.

Chief risks

"Gluten" is the term generally used to describe the toxic part of the protein found in wheat (gliadin), rye (secalin), and barley (hordein) that leads to celiac disease and dermatitis herpetiformis. You need to avoid gluten from these grains and other gluten-containing grains, such as triticale, spelt, Kamut, emmer, einkorn, and dinkle, all of which are closely related to wheat. Oats should also be avoided, not because of its gluten content but because of the high risk of cross-contamination with wheat, barley, or rye during food processing.

Wheat risks

Wheat grains are milled into many food products and processed into many ingredients — all to be avoided.

Milled wheat products

- Wheat bran
- Wheat germ
- Wheat flour
- Wheat starch
- Modified wheat starch

Wheat ingredients

- **Hydrolyzed wheat protein:** This processed wheat is typically used in seasonings or as a flavor enhancer in savory foods.
- **Modified wheat starch:** This starch has been altered through a chemical process to improve the texture of food products. When the modified starch is made from rice, corn, potato, or tapioca, it is gluten-free.
- **Dextrin made from wheat:** While rarely found in foods, dextrin is obtained from heating starch in the presence of moisture and acid. When made from wheat, it needs to be avoided.

Traditional foods made from wheat

- **Matzoh, matzoh meal:** Made from wheat flour, this flatbread is consumed around the time of Passover. In Europe, a few brands of matzoh are made from gluten-free ingredients and are considered kosher.
- **Seitan:** Also known as wheat meat, seitan is derived from wheat gluten and used in many vegetarian dishes.
- **Fu:** Used in a variety of Asian dishes, these thin sheets or thick cakes are derived from wheat gluten.
- **Tabbouleh:** This Middle Eastern dish is prepared with cracked wheat, parsley, onions, and tomatoes. In the gluten-free diet, the dish may be made with quinoa or millet as an alternative to cracked wheat.

Barley risks

Foods and ingredients derived from barley

- Barley flakes
- Barley flour
- Barley malt
- Malt flavoring
- Malt extract
- Malt syrup
- Malted milk
- Malt vinegar

Rye, Kamut, and spelt risks

Foods and ingredients derived from rye

- Rye flour
- Rye bread

Foods and ingredients derived from Kamut and spelt

- Kamut/spelt flours
- Kamut/spelt bread
- Kamut/spelt pasta
- Kamut/spelt pretzels and snacks

Oats risks

Foods and ingredients derived from oats

- Regular commercial oats
- Oatmeal
- Oat syrup
- Oat flour
- Oat bran

Tips for introducing pure, uncontaminated oats to your gluten-free diet:

- Wait to introduce pure, uncontaminated oats until you are stable on the gluten-free diet and until follow-up blood tests are within normal range.
- Once you introduce oats, make sure you follow up with your doctor 3 to 6 months later to monitor reactions and symptoms.
- When introducing oats, begin with small amounts, such as $\frac{1}{4}$ cup (75 mL) rolled oats once daily, at breakfast time. To ensure you can tolerate the amount of fiber, slowly increase this amount every week by $\frac{1}{4}$ cup until you reach $\frac{3}{4}$ cup.
- Do not forget to drink plenty of fluids while you are increasing the amount of fiber in your diet. Otherwise, you will experience symptoms of bloating, gas, and, possibly, constipation, which would be unrelated to celiac disease.

Did You Know?
Pure oats

Oat products may be highly contaminated with wheat, barley, and rye. However, pure, uncontaminated oats are currently available and, as the name indicates, pose very little risk to those with celiac disease. Nevertheless, there is no internationally acclaimed consensus on their safety. In North America, most of the celiac disease associations recommend introduction of pure oats in small quantities ($\frac{1}{2}$ to $\frac{3}{4}$ cup/125 to 175 mL dry rolled oats for adults and up to $\frac{1}{4}$ cup/60 mL for children) after 1 year of being on the gluten-free diet under medical supervision.

Suspect Foods

While some ingredients and foods are easily identified as safe or unsafe for the gluten-free diet, there is a gray area — that is, foods that you need to investigate when the ingredient label does not declare whether any of its components may be derived from gluten-containing grains. How well these suspect ingredients are listed on food labels varies from country to country. Take the time to call the manufacturer for full information on gluten content. Be sure any information you find on the Internet is from an authoritative source. Do your homework.

Modified food starch

If this product appears on a food label, ask yourself, What is the "food" in this starch? Is it wheat, corn, or potato? If the answer you receive from the manufacturer is wheat, avoid the food containing this ingredient. However, in many cases, it could be modified cornstarch, modified waxy maize starch, modified potato starch, or modified tapioca starch. All are acceptable in a gluten-free diet.

Modified Food Starch Labeling		
USA	**Canada**	**UK**
Currently the Food Allergen and Consumer Protection Act requires manufacturers to declare all top 8 allergens on the label. If wheat is used, it must appear on the label as "modified wheat starch" or "modified food starch (wheat)." Under the FDA's proposed new ruling on the use of the term "gluten-free," ingredients that have been processed to remove gluten, such as modified wheat starch, may be included in foods labeled "gluten-free" as long as the final concentration of gluten does not exceed 20 parts per million.	Currently there are no requirements for manufacturers to declare the source of modified food starch on the label. Consumers must contact the manufacturer to find out. New regulations are expected to mandate manufacturers to declare the source of gluten protein or modified gluten protein, including gluten protein fractions that are derived from wheat, barley, rye, spelt, Kamut, or triticale when they are present in foods or as part of food ingredients.	UK regulations require manufacturers to list all top 14 allergens and their derivatives on the label, including cereals containing gluten (wheat, rye, barley, oats, spelt, Kamut, or their hybridized strains) regardless of the amount used. If wheat is used, it must appear on the label as "modified wheat starch" or "modified food starch (contains wheat)."

Hydrolyzed plant/vegetable protein

This ingredient is widely used as a flavoring agent. Just as in the case of modified food starch, you need to ask yourself, What is the plant or vegetable source? If the answer is wheat, you need to avoid this. However, hydrolyzed soy protein and hydrolyzed corn protein are gluten-free.

Hydrolyzed Plant Protein Labeling

USA	Canada	UK
Currently the Food Allergen and Consumer Protection Act requires manufacturers to declare all top 8 allergens on the label. If wheat is used, it must appear on the label as "hydrolyzed wheat protein" or "hydrolyzed vegetable protein (wheat)." However, the Act does not require manufacturers to declare if ingredients are derived from barley or rye.	Currently there are no requirements for manufacturers to declare the source of hydrolyzed plant protein on the label. Consumers must contact the manufacturer to find out. New regulations are expected to mandate manufacturers to declare the source of gluten protein or modified gluten protein, including gluten protein fractions that are derived from wheat, barley, rye, spelt, Kamut, or triticale when they are present in foods or as part of food ingredients.	UK regulations require manufacturers to list all top 14 allergens on the label, including cereals containing gluten (wheat, rye, barley, oats, spelt, Kamut, or their hybridized strains) regardless of the amount used. If wheat is used, it must appear on the label as "hydrolyzed wheat protein" or "hydrolyzed vegetable protein (contains wheat)."

Seasonings

Blends of spices and herbs often use a carrier, such as wheat flour/wheat starch or hydrolyzed wheat protein. Seasonings may also contain salt, sugar, whey powder, and modified milk ingredients. Because of the high likelihood of wheat flour or wheat starch being used in seasonings, you need to always read the label or check with the manufacturer.

Glucose syrups

These sweeteners are derived from starch. In North America, the most common source of glucose syrup is cornstarch. However, in Europe wheat starch is more likely to be used. Data provided to the European Food Safety Association indicated that glucose syrups derived from wheat are highly refined and purified. In addition, numerous European clinical studies found no deleterious effects or increased inflammation in patients when daily consumption of wheat-based glucose syrups and maltodextrin was investigated.

Seasonings Labeling

USA	Canada	UK
Currently the Food Allergen and Consumer Protection Act requires manufacturers to declare all top 8 allergens on the label. If wheat is used, it must appear on the label as "seasonings (wheat)." However, the Act does not require manufacturers to declare if ingredients are derived from barley or rye.	Currently there are no requirements for manufacturers to declare any gluten-containing ingredients. Consumers must contact the manufacturer to find out. New regulations are expected to mandate manufacturers to declare the source of gluten protein or modified gluten protein, including gluten protein fractions that are derived from wheat, barley, rye, spelt, Kamut, or triticale when they are present in foods or as part of food ingredients.	UK regulations require manufacturers to list all top 14 allergens on the label, including cereals containing gluten (wheat, rye, barley, oats, spelt, Kamut, or their hybridized strains) regardless of the amount used. For example, "seasoning (salt, hydrolyzed wheat protein, black pepper)."

Glucose Syrups Labeling

USA	Canada	UK
Currently, for FDA-regulated foods, if glucose syrup is derived from wheat, the word "wheat" must be stated on the label. However, under the FDA's proposed ruling on the term "gluten-free," ingredients that have been processed to remove gluten may be included as ingredients in foods labeled "gluten-free" as long as their use does not exceed 20 parts per million or more of gluten.	Currently there are no requirements for manufacturers to declare the source of the starch used to produce glucose syrups. New regulations are expected to mandate manufacturers to declare the source of gluten protein or modified gluten protein, including gluten protein fractions that are derived from wheat, barley, rye, spelt, Kamut, or triticale when they are present in foods or as part of food ingredients.	According to the latest amended legislation, glucose syrups derived from wheat or barley, including dextrose, are exempt from allergen labeling, as evidence has shown that processing has removed the allergenic factor.

Foods under investigation

Some processed foods are under study to determine their gluten content. Until there is scientific evidence to prove they are gluten-free, it is probably best to avoid them.

Rice syrup

This sweetener is derived by culturing cooked whole-grain brown rice with enzymes to break down the starches, then straining off the liquid and cooking it until the desired consistency is reached. The final product is more slowly absorbed into the bloodstream because it carries a high soluble fiber content and protein from the whole grain. It is also more nutritious because it is a source of vitamins and minerals. The enzymes typically used in making rice syrup are fungal or bacterial in nature, but a few companies still use barley enzymes in the manufacturing of these types of syrups. Brown rice syrups are currently being tested to find out whether they contain significant amounts of residual gluten.

Smoke flavoring

This ingredient is another exception to the flavoring category. It has recently been found that some smoke flavoring contains wheat flour as a stabilizer. For this reason, it is extremely important to check the label every time.

Safe Foods

There are some food ingredients you need not worry about regardless of their origin. You can eat them without fear of aggravating symptoms of celiac disease.

Spices

Individual spices, such as cayenne pepper, paprika, allspice, and cinnamon, do not contain flour or starch and are gluten-free. Individual herbs, such as thyme, sage, oregano, and mint, are also gluten-free. And in 99% of cases, spice mixtures do not contain flour or starch and are gluten-free. However, that 1% has caused many individuals with celiac disease to shun spices.

If you are very concerned about the safety of spices, check with the manufacturer. There is no need to be afraid of spices — they enhance the taste of your meals, allow you to explore different cuisines, and provide an excellent source of antioxidants.

Spices Labeling

USA	Canada	UK
Currently the Food Allergen and Consumer Protection Act requires manufacturers to declare all top 8 allergens on the label. If wheat is used, it must appear on the label as "spices (wheat)." However, the Act does not require manufacturers to declare if ingredients are derived from barley or rye.	Spice mixtures, herb mixtures, and seasonings are exempt from ingredient declaration. New regulations are expected to mandate manufacturers to declare the source of gluten protein or modified gluten protein, including gluten protein fractions that are derived from wheat, barley, rye, spelt, Kamut, or triticale when they are present in foods or as part of food ingredients.	UK regulations mandate manufacturers to list all top 14 allergens on the label, including cereals containing gluten (wheat, rye, barley, oats, spelt, Kamut, or their hybridized strains). Spices, as with all foods sold prepacked within the UK, must be in compliance with these labeling regulations.

Maltodextrin

Maltodextrin is most often made from corn, potato, or rice starch. It is used as a bulking agent or fat replacer in a variety of low-fat products such as dairy products, nutritional beverages, jams, margarines, and some meat products. While it may rarely be derived from wheat, maltodextrin is so highly refined and filtered that results from one of the most sensitive scientifically validated gluten-detection tests indicated no significant amount of residual gluten in wheat-based maltodextrin.

Maltitol

This is a sugar substitute commonly found in chewing gum and many other sugar-free products. It is a derivative of corn syrup.

Food coloring

Food colorings are chemically derived and do not contain gluten. There have been some reported reactions to tartrazine — the yellow color in some candies — but this is unrelated to gluten. Colors are used in very small concentrations in food product formulations — up to 0.1% — and this is why you will find them listed at the end of the ingredient list.

Flavorings

Natural and artificial flavorings seldom use gluten-containing ingredients in their formulations. In most foods, flavors make up less than 1% of the recipe. When gluten-containing ingredients are used in flavorings, usually one of two ingredients may be declared: barley malt/malt flavoring or hydrolyzed wheat protein. As both are sources of allergens, they are almost always declared on the label. For these reasons, most experts agree that there is no need to restrict natural and artificial flavors in the gluten-free diet.

Flavorings Labeling		
USA	**Canada**	**UK**
Currently the Food Allergen and Consumer Protection Act requires manufacturers to declare all top 8 allergens on the label, including wheat but not barley or rye. If flavors are derived from barley, they will most likely be listed as "malt flavoring" on the food label. If hydrolyzed protein is used as a flavor enhancer, the source of the allergen must be declared and not hidden under the term "flavor."	Flavors, when used as ingredients in other foods, are exempt from ingredient declaration, with the exception of salt, glutamic acid, MSG, hydrolyzed plant protein, aspartame, and potassium chloride. New regulations are expected to mandate manufacturers to declare the source of gluten protein or modified gluten protein, including gluten protein fractions that are derived from wheat, barley, rye, spelt, Kamut, or triticale when they are present in foods or as part of food ingredients.	UK regulations mandate manufacturers to list all top 14 allergens on the label, including cereals containing gluten (wheat, rye, barley, oats, spelt, Kamut, or their hybridized strains). Flavorings, as with all foods sold prepacked within the UK, must be in compliance with these labeling regulations.

For further information on allergen labelling regulations, visit the following websites:

1. For the U.S. FDA's Food Allergen Labeling and Consumer Protection Act of 2004: www.fda.gov/Food/LabelingNutrition/FoodAllergensLabeling/default.htm.
2. For Canada's Food and Drug Act Regulations: http://laws.justice.gc.ca/en/showtdm/cr/C.R.C.-c.870.
3. For Health Canada's Enhanced Labelling for Food Allergen and Gluten Sources and Added Sulphites: www.hc-sc.gc.ca/fn-an/label-etiquet/allergen/.
4. For the U.K. Food Standards Agency's Food Allergen Labelling: www.food.gov.uk/safereating/allergyintol/label/.

Shopping for Gluten-Free Groceries

The gluten-free diet presents a great opportunity to reinvent the way you shop and to go back to the roots of healthy eating. Most patients I have met in my practice feel much better about the way they eat when they acknowledge and embrace the fact that they have to deal with celiac disease and the only way to treat it is by eating a gluten-free diet. They shop differently, no longer relying on processed foods. They find themselves shopping along the perimeter of the grocery store. One by one, fresh fruits and vegetables and fresh meats/poultry/fish, followed by dairy/eggs/cheese, become their new staples.

Shopping tips

Celiac disease or not, here are some rules of thumb for healthy shopping:

1. **Buy fresh food!** What could be healthier and more wholesome? The beauty of the gluten-free diet is that most fresh foods are also gluten-free. Fruits, vegetables, fresh meats, poultry, seafood, dairy, legumes, and fruit juices are the healthiest of foods and also gluten-free. Remember how your parents and grandparents used to cook? Fresh and simple.

2. **Always shop the perimeter of the store first.** The less you find yourself in the center aisles, the easier and healthier your trip to the grocery store will be.

3. **Shop with a list.** Save time, money, and empty calories by sticking to what you know you need. This will prevent you from wandering toward the snacks aisle.

4. **Speak up at the deli counter.** If you are buying deli meat, ensure against gluten contamination by asking that the blade be cleaned before the deli clerk slices your order. Be proactive and ensure that the brands of deli meats you choose are gluten-free.

5. **Do not shop on an empty stomach.** Have a snack before you head out shopping. This will make you less vulnerable to buying calorie-rich snacks like potato chips and chocolate bars — yes, many of these are gluten-free! If you can't have a meal, plan to bring along a snack, such as a piece of fruit and a few almonds, walnuts, or soy nuts.

6. **Stock up on frozen fruits and vegetables.** Believe it or not, frozen fruits and veggies are just as healthy, if not healthier, than fresh ones! Often they are ripe and flash-frozen at the source, meaning that nutrients and antioxidants are preserved. You can easily incorporate vegetables in soups, quiches, and casseroles. Fruits can easily be served over gluten-free waffles or pancakes, incorporated into smoothies, or mixed in with yogurt or ice cream. When the season's over for berries, buy frozen ones without added sugars to get a taste of summer!

7. **Embrace the mighty bean.** Most brands of regular canned beans are not only gluten-free but also filling, nutritious, and delicious. A cup of cooked beans is an excellent source of fiber (15 grams), folate, iron, and calcium. Beans have been linked to lowering cholesterol, reducing plaque in patients with fatty plaques in their arteries, and improving insulin resistance.

8. **Look for fiber.** Lack of fiber leads to constipation and is a challenge when you're following the gluten-free diet. Introducing too much fiber too quickly can cause gastrointestinal discomfort, such as gas, bloating, and cramping. Take it easy as you introduce or increase servings of quinoa, corn, pure oats, and other gluten-free alternatives to wheat.

9. **Dress up your morning cereal.** You don't need to limit yourself to plain cream of rice. Why not add some fresh or frozen fruit, raisins, plain roasted almond slivers, walnuts, pumpkin seeds, sunflower seeds, ground flax seeds, or chia seeds? Make your own trail mix, keep it in a well-sealed wide-mouth jar, and add a tablespoon or two to your cereal or eat $1/4$ cup (60 mL) for an afternoon snack on the go.

10. **Buy plain yogurt and flavor it at home.** For many of my patients, the taste of plain yogurt just doesn't cut it. However, the commercial brands almost always have too much sugar and empty calories. Consider adding a teaspoon (5 mL) of honey or jam to plain yogurt along with your favorite frozen berries and some cinnamon or nutmeg. It will still be delicious, and you will save both calories and money.

11. **Try delicious gluten-free baked items.** Wheat is not the only grain with nutritional properties. Plenty of alternative grains are delicious and nutritious!

Aisle-by-Aisle Guide

Here is a guide to gluten-free foods that you will find in each section and along the aisles of a typical grocery store. Foods are rated as Enjoy, Suspect, or Avoid:

- **Enjoy** these foods without risk of gluten.
- **Suspect** these foods by reading the label closely or checking with the manufacturer when you get home.
- **Avoid** these foods because they contain gluten.

You can use this guide as a shopping list. Just check off what you need and power up the shopping cart.

Produce

Produce section

Enjoy
- Whole fresh fruits
- Whole fresh vegetables
- Freshly cut ready-to-eat fruits
- Freshly cut ready-to-eat vegetables
- Packaged salads

Suspect
- Some dried fruits (for example, dates)
- Fruits prepared in sauce

Dairy

Dairy, dairy alternatives, and eggs section

Enjoy
- Milk
- Buttermilk
- Cream
- Butter
- Margarine
- Chocolate milk
- Cottage cheese
- Hard aged cheeses (Cheddar cheese, Swiss cheese, mozzarella, Havarti, Monterey Jack, Parmesan, Asiago, Gouda, Lappi)
- Processed cheese slices
- Cottage cheese
- Soft cheese (blue cheese, Brie, Stilton, Oka)
- Fresh eggs

- Plain liquid egg products
- Plain tofu
- Soy-based butter, vegetable shortening

Suspect
- Flavored yogurts (may contain gluten-containing ingredients such as granola and oats)
- Frozen yogurts (cookies 'n' cream or cookie dough may contain gluten ingredients)
- Products containing malt flavoring
- Seasoned shredded cheese (may contain hydrolyzed wheat protein)
- Cheese sauces (may contain wheat starch/flour or hydrolyzed wheat protein)
- Cheese spreads
- Soy-based dairy products (puddings, cream cheese, flavored Cheddar/mozzarella, yogurt); while most are gluten-free, ensure that no gluten-containing ingredients such as brewer's yeast, malt extract, or wheat starch are used.
- Seasoned liquid egg products
- Soy milk (may contain barley malt, barley enzymes, or wheat flour)
- Soy-based ice cream
- Flavored cream cheese
- Soy-based meats (may contain hydrolyzed wheat protein or wheat flour)
- Rice-based dairy alternatives (watch for gluten-containing ingredients such as wheat starch and brewer's yeast)

Avoid
- Malted milk
- Lactose-free coffee whitener
- Tofu seasoned with soy sauce or teriyaki sauce (contains wheat)

Deli section

Deli

Enjoy
- Gluten-free deli meats: turkey breast, chicken breast, roast beef, pastrami, prosciutto

Suspect
- Bacon (most brands of bacon are gluten-free, but some may contain soy sauce made with wheat)
- Ham (most hams are gluten-free, but, rarely, some may contain wheat starch, wheat flour, or soy sauce)
- Salami (most is gluten-free, but some may contain hydrolyzed wheat protein)

- Kielbasa sausage (may contain hydrolyzed wheat protein or wheat flour/starch)
- Wieners or frankfurters (may contain hydrolyzed wheat protein or wheat flour/starch)
- Liver pâté (may contain wheat flour or wheat starch)

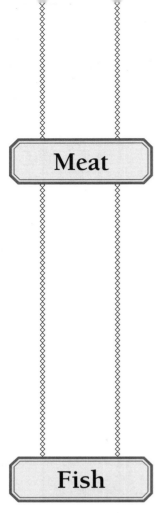

Meat section

Enjoy
- All fresh lean cuts of beef, lamb, veal, pork
- All fresh poultry (chicken, turkey)

Suspect
- Sausages (may contain ingredients made from hydrolyzed wheat protein or wheat flour/starch)
- Meatballs (may contain bread crumbs as part of the recipe)
- Dried meats such as beef jerky (may contain soy sauce or wheat flour)
- Frozen hamburgers (may contain wheat starch or hydrolyzed wheat protein)

Avoid
- Frozen turkeys and pork roasts filled with bread stuffing
- Seasoned frozen turkeys and chicken breasts (may contain hydrolyzed wheat protein)

Fish Section

Enjoy
- All fresh or frozen fish
- All fresh or frozen real seafood: shrimp, scallops, crab, lobster, clams, mussels
- Oysters
- Canned tuna in water or oil
- Canned sardines in water or oil

Suspect
- Smoked fish such as salmon (smoke flavoring may contain gluten)
- Canned tuna in vegetable broth (may contain hydrolyzed wheat protein)
- Canned sardines in vegetable broth (may contain hydrolyzed wheat protein)
- Imitation crabmeat, also known as surimi (may contain wheat starch)

Avoid
- Breaded fish sticks
- Breaded/battered shrimp
- Seasoned fish in pouches

Aisle 1

Breakfast Cereals, Hot Cereal, Jam, Peanut Butter, Canned Fruit, Syrups

Enjoy
- Gluten-free cold cereals: corn, amaranth, quinoa, rice, and flax cereal
- Gluten-free granola cereal
- Hot cereals: cream of buckwheat, quinoa flakes, cream of brown rice, millet grits, cornmeal, mixed hot cereal made with gluten-free grits (quinoa, corn, amaranth)
- Jam
- Marmalade
- Seed butters (sesame, sunflower, pumpkin seeds)
- Canned fruit

Suspect
- Corn cereals (may contain barley malt or malt flavoring not listed as an ingredient)
- Rice cereals (may contain barley malt or malt flavoring not listed as an ingredient)
- Cereals sweetened with rice malt or rice syrup (watch for barley enzymes used in the manufacturing process)
- Canned fruit sauce
- Peanut butter (most brands are gluten-free, but some may use wheat germ)
- Nut butters (most brands are gluten-free, but some may use wheat germ)

Avoid
- Cold breakfast cereals containing ingredients derived from wheat, barley, rye, triticale, Kamut, spelt, einkorn, or emmer
- Regular oatmeal, oat bran, steel-cut oats, large-flake oats (high risk of cross-contamination with gluten-containing grains)
- Hot cereals containing ingredients derived from wheat, barley, rye, triticale, Kamut, spelt, einkorn, emmer, or commercial oats
- Regular granola bars made with commercial oats and other gluten-containing ingredients

Aisle 2

Cookies, Confectionery, Crackers, Potato Chips, Snacks, Popcorn

Enjoy
- Gluten-free cookies
- Gluten-free crackers
- Plain or salted popcorn
- Rice cakes
- Corn tortilla chips

Suspect

- Chocolate: ensure no malt flavoring
- Chocolate bars: watch for gluten-containing ingredients
- Seasoned potato chips: watch for hydrolyzed wheat protein
- Seasoned taco chips
- Seasoned nuts, soynuts: watch for wheat starch and soy sauce containing wheat
- Seasoned rice cakes: watch for gluten-containing ingredients

Avoid

- Trail mixes
- Licorice candy
- Nuts or seeds mixes from the bulk section
- Candy made with gluten-containing ingredients

Aisle 3

Spices, Flour, Baking Ingredients, Sugar

Enjoy

- Individual spices (e.g., cinnamon, pepper, cloves, allspice, ginger, paprika)
- Individual herbs (e.g., thyme, basil, sage, savory)
- Amaranth flour
- Arrowroot flour (not to be confused with Arrowroot biscuits, made with wheat flour and arrowroot flour)
- Corn flour
- Cornmeal
- Corn bran
- Cornstarch
- Potato starch
- Quinoa flour
- Whole flax seeds
- Ground flax seeds (flaxseed meal)
- Millet flour and grits
- Legume flour (e.g., fava, gram, besan, garbanzo or chickpea, lentil)
- Sorghum flour
- Brown rice flour
- Whole-grain rice flour
- Glutinous rice flour
- Tapioca flour (manioc or cassava root powder)
- Indian rice grass
- Inulin (dietary fiber found in artichokes, leeks, and chicory root)
- Psyllium husks
- Nut flours (almond, hazelnut, chestnut)
- Potato flour

- Pure, uncontaminated (wheat-free, gluten-free) oat flour, oat bran
- Chia seeds (oil seeds derived from an ancient plant species belonging to the mint family Chia, grown in Peru)
- Sago (starchy food derived from palm trees)
- Soy flour
- Teff flour
- Taro flour
- Sweet potato flour
- Gluten-free pancake mixes
- Gluten-free bread mixes
- Baking soda
- Active dry yeast
- Baker's yeast
- Nutritional yeast
- Xanthan gum
- Guar gum
- Vanilla extract (pure or artificial)
- Rum extract
- Food coloring
- Carob chips
- Pure cocoa powder
- Cream of tartar
- Shredded coconut
- Baking chocolate
- Chocolate chips
- Carob bean "chocolate"
- Corn syrup
- Blackstrap molasses
- Maple syrup
- White or brown sugar
- Raw sugar
- Agave nectar
- Confectioners' (icing) sugar

Did You Know?
Gluten-free flours

Gluten-free flours, such as buckwheat, corn, legume, and even some rice flours, have been reported to contain levels of gluten because of cross-contamination. Always contact the manufacturing company to ensure that the milling and packaging of these flours is done in a designated gluten-free area to minimize the risk of accidently ingesting gluten.

Suspect

- Spice mixtures (while spices are gluten-free, in one case the spice blend contained wheat flour as part of the formulation, which does not reflect food industry trends)
- Buckwheat flour (may sometimes be mixed with wheat flour in a product, and there is a high likelihood of cross-contamination)

- Baking powder (generally made with cornstarch, but, rarely, some may contain wheat starch)
- Icing mixes and frosting (may contain wheat starch or wheat flour)

Avoid
- Atta and chapatti flour (low-gluten wheat flour used to make chapatti flatbreads, a specialty of Indian cuisine)
- Wheat flour
- Wheat starch
- Wheat germ
- Semolina flour
- Durum wheat flour
- Regular cake and pancake mixes
- Buckwheat pancake mixes containing wheat flour
- Ice cream cones and wafers made from wheat flour

Aisle 4

Oils, Vinegars, Sauces, Salad Dressings, Condiments

Enjoy
- All vegetable oils
- Distilled vinegars (distilled white, cider, apple, balsamic, wine vinegar)
- Mustard bran
- Mustard flour
- Most pickles
- Ketchup
- Most relish
- Olives
- Tomato paste
- Hot sauce
- Gluten-free soy sauce
- Real bacon bits
- Roasted red peppers
- Roasted artichokes
- Roasted tomatoes

Suspect
- Cooking sauces (may contain wheat starch, modified wheat starch, or hydrolyzed wheat protein)
- Imitation bacon bits (may contain hydrolyzed wheat protein)
- Prepared mustard (some specialty mustards may contain wheat flour)
- Prepared mustard flour (may contain wheat starch or wheat flour)
- Mustard pickles (may contain wheat starch or wheat flour)

Did You Know?
Vinegar choices

The majority of rice vinegars are distilled and gluten-free. However, a small number of examples have revealed labeling inaccuracies in products made in Asia (China, Hong Kong, Korea). Some of you will find rice vinegar bottles listing wheat as an ingredient or "rice vinegar (wheat)." Wheat may be a used in the fermentation process of the bacterial cultures used to make the vinegar. However, the risk of gluten being present in the vinegar is very small. When the vinegar is distilled, the product is gluten-free regardless of the source or gluten-containing ingredients that may be used in the fermentation process.

- Creamy salad dressings (e.g., creamy Caesar, ranch, Thousand Island; may contain wheat starch or wheat flour)
- Barbecue sauce (may contain malt vinegar)
- Worcestershire sauce (may contain malt vinegar)
- Peanut sauce (may contain wheat flour or wheat starch)
- Textured vegetable protein (may contain wheat starch or hydrolyzed wheat protein)

Avoid
- Malt vinegar (made from barley and other grains; not distilled)
- Soy sauce (usually contains wheat, but some brands of gluten-free soy sauce are available)
- Tamari sauce (contains wheat, but some brands of gluten-free tamari sauce are available)
- Teriyaki sauce containing soy sauce
- Gravy containing wheat flour
- Creamy salad dressings containing wheat flour or wheat starch
- Suet

Aisle 5

Aisle 5

Soup, Canned Vegetables, Dried and Canned Beans, Pasta, Pasta Sauce, Mexican Foods, Rice

Enjoy
- All dried beans, lentils, and pulses
- All dried peas
- Regular canned beans, lentils, peas, pulses
- Pasta made from rice, quinoa, soy, beans, lentils, or potato
- Soup broth labeled "gluten-free"
- Ready-to-eat soups made with "gluten-free" ingredients
- Corn tortilla chips
- Corn tacos

Suspect
- Buckwheat noodles: ensure that pure buckwheat flour is used
- Seasoned rice mixtures (e.g., chicken wild rice, chicken with vegetables)
- Soup mixes: watch for hydrolyzed wheat protein and wheat starch
- Bean soup mixes that include seasonings
- Canned soup
- Bouillon cubes
- Some brands of baked beans
- Soft tortillas made with corn flour (ensure that the corn flour is gluten-free)
- Salsa (most brands are gluten-free, but some may use smoke flavoring containing wheat starch)

- Guacamole
- Cheese sauces
- Creamy pasta sauces (ensure no wheat flour or wheat starch)
- Tomato-based pasta sauces (most are gluten-free, but check for the presence of modified food starch made from wheat)

Avoid
- Couscous
- Orzo
- Whole wheat pasta
- Multigrain pasta
- Durum semolina pasta
- Udon noodles
- Soft tortillas made with a combination of corn and wheat flours
- Commercial powdered mashed potatoes made with wheat starch/wheat flour
- Scalloped potatoes containing wheat flour

Aisle 6

Aisle 6

Water, Soft Drinks, Sports Drinks, Fruit Juice

Enjoy
- Water
- Flavored water
- Fresh fruit juices
- Shelf-stable juices
- Soft drinks
- Tea
- Coffee (dried, instant, or ground)
- Wine
- Bourbon
- Gin
- Port
- Rye whisky
- Scotch whisky
- Vodka
- Liqueurs

Suspect
- Sports drinks (ensure that gluten-free ingredients are used)
- Flavored herbal teas (ensure that no malt or malt flavoring is used)
- Flavored coffee (ensure that no malt or malt flavoring is used)
- Chocolate drinks
- Flavored alcohol coolers
- Flavored vodka mixes (e.g., Bloody Mary)

Avoid
- Malted drinks
- Coffee substitutes made with barley malt
- Beer (lager, ale, porter, stout)

Aisle 7

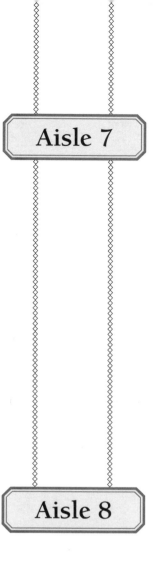

Frozen Fruits, Frozen Vegetables, Frozen Deserts

Enjoy
- Frozen fruits (plain)
- Frozen vegetables and vegetable mixes (plain)
- Frozen gluten-free foods (gluten-free pizza, gluten-free chili, etc.)

Suspect
- Frozen french fries (wheat starch or hydrolyzed wheat protein may be used in the seasoning)
- Restaurant-made frozen french fries
- Deep-fried foods made in the same fryer (ensure no cross-contamination with other battered foods by checking with the manufacturer)
- Seasoned frozen vegetables

Avoid
- Battered frozen vegetables
- Frozen pies, pizza
- Frozen pasta dishes

Aisle 8

Shampoo, Dental Care, Deodorant, Soap, Cosmetics

Cosmetics and toiletries containing wheat do not pose a risk to those with celiac disease unless they are ingested. Sometimes those who suffer from dermatitis herpetiformis report that their symptoms seem to worsen when they apply gluten-containing creams, deodorants, and shampoos to the skin and scalp. If this happens, see your doctor. Your skin may simply be sensitive to specific chemicals or fragrances.

Lipstick, lip balm, and lip gloss are three products that you should check for gluten-containing ingredients. Most experts agree, however, that the amount of gluten in these products is very small and the amount you might ingest should be even smaller. Toothpastes and mouthwash products are typically gluten-free, but it is always safer to check with the manufacturer.

Gluten-Proofing the Kitchen

Now that you've brought home a few bags of gluten-free groceries, you will need to organize your pantry and refrigerator to preserve these foods and to prevent cross-contamination with any gluten-containing foods your family may still be eating. Taking on the gluten-free diet can prompt a major overhaul of your kitchen. If you are the only person with celiac disease in the household, you need to decide whether the family is going gluten-free or if you will be the only one following the diet. If you have children and they have not yet been diagnosed, you would be best not to put them on the gluten-free diet 100% of the time, since doing so could mask or delay the eventual diagnosis. Most patients find a balance, choosing to keep some packaged gluten-containing foods for the rest of the family but making the main dishes, desserts, and breads gluten-free. Most of the time nobody notices the difference because most gluten-free meals are delicious and easy to make.

Guide to gluten-proofing

Whatever you decide, you will need to prevent gluten contamination of gluten-free foods. Here is a guide to gluten-proofing your kitchen.

Pantry

1. **Clean out your pantry cupboard** and divide the foods you have into two groups:

   - **Keepers:** Foods that are safe to eat, such as canned tuna, salmon, or real crabmeat, canned sardines, beans (canned or dry), rice, pure spices, canned vegetables, canned fruit, tomato-based pasta sauce (check for gluten first), honey, peanut butter, rice vermicelli or rice paper, chili sauce, oil, vinegars (except malt vinegar).

   - **Giveaways:** Foods you'll have give away to relatives, friends, or neighbors. Use this opportunity as an ice-breaker for letting close relatives and friends know about your new diagnosis. These foods include breads, tortillas, crackers made from gluten-containing flours, cold and hot cereals, flours you used for baking, ready-made baking mixes, regular pasta, couscous, scalloped potatoes, seasoned rice mixes, other gluten-containing grains (wheat berries, barley, rye, oats, spelt, Kamut, triticale), cornmeal not labeled gluten-free, Worcestershire sauce, and barbecue sauce made with malt vinegar.

2. Now stock the pantry with foods to share with the rest of your family. Guess what? There are many foods that are gluten-free and delicious, including snack foods (gluten-free potato chips, cookies, corn chips, nuts, seeds, cheesy snacks, flavored rice cakes, chocolate bars).

3. Dedicate a pantry shelf to foods that are gluten-free and that will be for your use only.

Refrigerator

1. Again, sort out the keepers from the giveaways.

   - **Keepers:** milk, chocolate milk (ensure that no malt ingredients are used), individual servings of yogurt, juice, soy milk (check if it is gluten-free), squeezable bottles of plain mustard, ketchup and mayonnaise, butter, oil-based salad dressings (ensure that they are gluten-free).

   - **Giveaways:** While a lot of refrigerated foods are perishable, if there are products you used to enjoy and can take over to a relative's or friend's house, you may avoid having to throw them away.

2. Restock with gluten-free foods and label them with your own name: butter or margarine, peanut/nut/seed butter jars, jars of jam, jelly, fruit butters, or honey (you may purchase the squeezable kind of bottle); any other jars of condiments that people other than yourself use.

Appliances

1. **Buy a new toaster for gluten-free toast.** Don't be tempted to wash an existing toaster or divide a 4-slot toaster into "gluten" and "gluten-free" sides. It's only a toaster. Why sabotage all the other efforts you are making to maintain a gluten-free diet for the cost of a toaster?

2. **Use a toaster oven as an alternative.** The gluten-containing and gluten-free foods can be separated by a sheet of aluminum foil or a clean dish.

Counters

Before starting meal preparation or whenever you prepare your own snacks or meals, make sure you clean the counters to avoid the risk of contaminating your food because another member of your household may have left crumbs of bread, crackers, or cookies on that counter.

Did You Know?
Separate Tools

Keep a separate cutting board for foods containing gluten. Also purchase a separate mesh colander for straining your gluten-free pasta and other foods.

Substitutes for Gluten-Containing Grains

There is a wide selection of foods that can be used instead of gluten-containing products, including a good variety of grains, beans, and seeds. Many people find these substitutes more appealing than standard wheat, barley, and rye grains and flours. Give them all a try — you may find a new favorite food and never regret avoiding gluten.

Gluten-free grains, seeds, and beans

Among gluten-free grains and seeds are rice (japonica red, wild, brown, black), amaranth, arrowroot, flax, millet, quinoa, sorghum, teff, bean flour, chestnut flour, corn starch, potato starch, and tapioca starch.

Amaranth

Amaranth is a broadleaf plant that develops brilliantly colored grain heads producing thousands of tiny seeds. Amaranth was a major food of the Aztecs and earlier American cultures. Amaranth seeds are unusually high in protein for a non-legume, running to around 14% to 16% protein. Even better, the protein is well balanced in amino acids, and especially high in lysine, an amino acid most grains are deficient in (legumes also have high lysine). A traditional use of amaranth is to mix popped amaranth with a sweet, sticky foodstuff, such as molasses or honey, to make a type of snack bar or snack cake (not unlike a granola bar or crispy rice bar). The whole seed is sometimes used in a type of porridge or as a condiment on other foods. The ground flour is made into a variety of baked breads. Amaranth is very high in iron, magnesium, and manganese content.

Culinary profile

Whole-grain amaranth has a nutty flavor. The seeds may be ground into flour and used in cereal or for making bread or muffins. You may find puffed amaranth sold as a cold cereal or as a side dish in supermarkets, but amaranth flour is typically found in specialty food stores or health food stores.

Cooking with amaranth

Whole-grain amaranth may cook in as little as 20 to 25 minutes when boiled in water, gluten-free stock, juice, or coconut milk, in a ratio of 1 part grain to 3 parts liquid.

You may turn ready-to-eat puffed amaranth into a hot cereal or side dish by adding the desired amount of liquid and mixing. Use a 1:1 ratio (1 part puffed amaranth to 1 part liquid).

Storing

Store amaranth in a cool, dry area in a sealed glass or plastic container to prevent it from going rancid. No refrigeration is needed.

Nutritional profile

Amaranth grain, cooked, 1/2 cup (125 g)	Values	% of Daily Value
Calories (kcal)	120	—
Fat (g)	1.58	2.4
Protein (g)	3.8	7.6
Carbohydrates (g)	18.7	6.2
Fiber (g)	2.1	8.4
Folate (mcg)	22.0	5.5
Calcium (mg)	47.0	4.7
Iron (mg)	2.10	12.0
Magnesium (mg)	65.0	16.0
Manganese (mg)	0.85	43.0
(Source: Food Processor SQL 2009 edition)		

Arrowroot

Arrowroot is a tropical tuber (*Maranta arundinacea*) originating in the West Indies and South America but now widely cultivated throughout Asia, Africa, and the Pacific islands. It is also known as cassava or manioc, particularly in South America.

Culinary profile

Arrowroot in its true form, as grown in the West Indies, can be eaten raw, roasted, or boiled. However, arrowroot is most widely used as a starch. When pulverized into a fine-textured powder, arrowroot is suitable for using as a thickener in soups, sauces, gravies, and puddings in lieu of wheat flour. When dissolved, the starch is translucent and glossy and provides a nice glazing effect. Arrowroot flour or starch is also suitable for baking breads, cookies, and pastries to promote better binding. The British and early Americans used arrowroot flour in cookie recipes.

Cooking with arrowroot

Pure arrowroot powder is light and white, and odorless until cooked. It then becomes translucent and glossy and feels very much like cornstarch. You may use 3 tablespoons (45 mL) of powder to 1 cup (250 mL) water. Place arrowroot powder in a saucepan, mix slowly with water until smooth, and stir over medium-high heat until the gel boils and clears. You may use arrowroot instead of wheat flour to thicken sauces, soups, and gravies or to make pudding.

Storing

Store arrowroot in a cool, dark place in a container or jar with a tight-fitting lid. Do not freeze or refrigerate.

Nutritional profile		
Arrowroot starch, ¾ cup (100 g)	Values	% of Daily Value
Calories (kcal)	357	—
Fat (g)	0.1	0.15
Protein (g)	0.3	0.6
Carbohydrates (g)	88	29.4
Fiber (g)	3.4	13.6
Folate (mcg)	7.0	1.7
Calcium (mg)	40.0	4.0
Iron (mg)	0.33	1.8
Magnesium (mg)	3.0	0.8
Manganese (mg)	0.47	23.5
		(Source: Food Processor SQL 2009 edition)

Bean flours

The Leguminosae family is another group of plants whose seeds are nutritional powerhouses. Some of the most commonly used seeds, such as peanuts, peas, lentils, and beans, have been an important dietary staple for thousands of years. Unfortunately, beans are so closely associated with gas and bloating that many people avoid them altogether. The beauty of bean flours is that manufacturers pretreat dried peas and beans to reduce the flatulence effects, then grind them into flours. What's more, most beans and bean flours are inexpensive.

Culinary profile

There are many types of legume flours that may be used in gluten-free baking:

- fava bean flour
- chickpea flour
- white bean flour
- pinto bean flour
- pea flour
- whole bean flour

The bean flours add body and flavor as well as protein and fiber to rice flour mixes and other baking mixes, such as brownie mixes, all-purpose baking mixes, pancake mixes and bread mixes.

Cooking with bean flours

Bean flours combine well with other gluten-free flours, particularly brown rice and sorghum flours. They work well in baking recipes using molasses and brown sugar. Chickpea flour is popular in Middle Eastern cuisine, where it is a major ingredient of falafel and hummus recipes. Yellow and green pea flours keep baked products softer longer, improve dough made in bread machines, and reduce mixing times.

Storing bean flours

Store flours for up to 6 months in tightly-lidded containers in the refrigerator or for up to 1 year in the freezer.

Nutritional profile

Bean flours are higher in protein than any other plant-based or grain-based flour. They are also high in fiber and packed with calcium, iron, folate, zinc, potassium, magnesium, and B vitamins.

Buckwheat

While many people think of buckwheat as a cereal grain, it is actually a fruit seed. If it is not related to wheat, where does buckwheat derive its name from? The name is supposedly derived from the Dutch word *bockweit*, which means "beech wheat," reflecting buckwheat's beechnut-like shape and its wheat-like characteristics. Buckwheat is a broadleaf plant native to northern Asia and a relative of rhubarb and sorrel. The seeds are brown in color and roughly the size of a soybean, but irregularly shaped, with four triangular surfaces. Buckwheat flowers profusely, making it a favorite with beekeepers. Buckwheat honey is a delicious treat.

Don't let the "wheat" in buckwheat keep you away from this seed — it is gluten-free! Buckwheat flour is used most often in pancakes or waffles. Buckwheat bran is extremely nutritious, high in fiber, protein, iron, riboflavin, niacin, and many antioxidants to help boost your immune system.

Culinary profile

Most buckwheat is ground into flour and used for a variety of foods, including noodles in Japan and pancakes and breakfast cereals in North America. Russians and Eastern Europeans make a wide range of foods with buckwheat.

Cooking with buckwheat

Roasted groats, also known as kasha, are cooked like rice and traditionally used as a filling for stuffed chicken, in soups, or as a side dish. Kasha has a robust, earthy flavor and can make a delicious addition to vegetable soups. Rinse the whole grains thoroughly under running water. To cook, add 1 part buckwheat to 2 parts boiling water or broth. After the liquid has returned to a boil, turn down the heat, cover, and simmer for about 30 minutes.

Buckwheat, 1 cup (250 mL)	Liquid	Cooking Time	Yield	Additional Info
Roasted groats, uncooked	2 cups (500 mL)	10 minutes + let stand for 5 minutes	2½ cups (625 mL)	
Cream of buckwheat	5 cups (1.25 L)	6–8 minutes	3 cups	May also be used as an infant cereal; once cooked, just add breast milk or formula.

Storing buckwheat

Keep buckwheat groats (kasha) in an airtight container and store in a cool, dry place for up to 1 year. Buckwheat flour can be stored in the refrigerator for several months.

Nutritional profile

Buckwheat's beneficial effects are due in part to its rich supply of flavonoids, particularly rutin. Rutin is a phytonutrient that enhances the action of antioxidants, such as vitamin C. It is responsible for buckwheat's claim to be protective against heart disease. Buckwheat is a very good source of manganese and a good source of magnesium and dietary fiber.

Nutritional profile		
Buckwheat, roasted, cooked, $3/4$ cup (100 g)	Values	% of Daily Value
Calories (kcal)	92	—
Fat (g)	0.62	1.0
Protein (g)	3.38	6.8
Carbohydrates (g)	20.0	6.7
Fiber (g)	3.0	10.0
Iron (mg)	0.8	4.0
Magnesium (mg)	51.0	13.0
Manganese (mg)	0.4	20.0
(Source: Food Processor SQL 2009 edition)		

Chestnut flour

Before corn was introduced to Italy from the New World, polenta was originally made from chestnut meal. Chestnut flour is more expensive than other gluten-free flours.

Culinary profile

This is a fine, sweet flour that is renowned for its delicate texture and sweet flavor. It is used most commonly in Italian artisanal baking and it imparts a distinct sweet and velvety mouth-feel.

Cooking with chestnut flour

Chestnut flour is used for making desserts, pastries, and artisanal breads. You may use it to replace 100% or partially substitute for the amount of wheat flour called for in cakes and muffins.

Storing chestnut flour

Because chestnuts have very little fat content, chestnut flour may last for 12 to 18 months when kept in a tightly lidded container in a dark, cool, dry place.

Nutritional profile		
Chestnut flour, 1 cup (100 g)	**Values**	**% of Daily Value**
Calories (kcal)	371	—
Fat (g)	3.67	8.0
Protein (g)	6.55	13.0
Carbohydrates (g)	78.0	7.0
Fiber (g)	9.2	33.0
Folate (mcg)	70.0	17.0
Calcium (mg)	35.0	3.0
Copper (mg)	0.51	25.0
Manganese (mg)	1.18	59.0
Molybdenum (mg)	25.9	39.3

(Source: www.chestnutgrowersinc.com)

Corn flour, corn masa and cornmeal

Corn is thought to have originated in Mexico or Central America and dates back almost 7,000 years. It has a strong mythological significance to the Mayan, Incan, and Aztec civilizations. In North America, corn is an extremely popular food. From the juicy, sweet field corn we savor during the summer to popcorn at the movies, corn flakes, and cornbread, this plant has so many uses! Corn grits are so popular in the Southern United States that the state of Georgia declared grits its official food in 2002.

However, some brands of corn flour or cornmeal may be contaminated with gluten-containing grains such as wheat or barley. Ensure that the brand you buy is free of contaminants.

Culinary profile

Corn kernels are processed into many different products:

- hominy (hulled corn kernels that have been stripped of the bran and germ)
- hominy grits (ground hominy)
- masa harina (flour made from hominy grits)
- stone-ground cornmeal (dried ground corn kernels)
- corn flour (finely ground cornmeal)
- cornstarch (white, flavorless, starchy powder used as a thickening agent)

Cooking with corn

Hominy grits are widely used in Southern American cooking to make a porridge served either as a breakfast meal or as a side dish mixed with vegetables. Cornmeal is the basis for polenta, an Italian tradition that may be served as a side dish or on its own with a variety of sauces. Cornmeal may also be incorporated into batters or used as a coating for frying fish or schnitzel. Corn flour makes delicious muffins, pie crusts, and breads.

Cornmeal, 1 cup (250 mL)	Liquid	Cooking Time	Yield	Additional Info
Coarse, uncooked	4½ cups (1.125 L)	25–30 minutes	3½ cups (875 mL)	For polenta you need to stir frequently to avoid clumping and to allow the liquid to incorporate into the polenta mix.

Storing corn flour or cornmeal

If you are using cornmeal often, you may store it in a tightly lidded container in a cool, dark, dry place for up to 1 month. If you would like it to last longer, keep it in an airtight container in the refrigerator for up to 2 months or in the freezer for up to 6 months.

Nutritional profile

Cornmeal, ¾ cup (100 g)	Values	% of Daily Value
Calories (kcal)	362	—
Fat (g)	3.6	5.5
Protein (g)	8.12	16.0
Carbohydrates (g)	77.0	26.0
Fiber (g)	7.3	29.0
Vitamin B_1 – thiamin (mg)	0.4	26.0
Vitamin B_2 – riboflavin (mg)	0.2	12.0
Vitamin B_3 – niacin (mg)	3.6	18.0
Vitamin B_6 (mg)	0.3	15.2
Chromium (mcg)	32.8	27.0
Iron (mg)	3.45	19.0
Magnesium (mg)	127.0	31.75
Manganese (mg)	0.5	25.0
Molybdenum (mcg)	56	74.7
Phosphorus (mg)	241	24.0
Selenium (mcg)	15.5	22.0
	(Source: Food Processor SQL 2009 edition)	

Flax

Flax comes from a blue-flowered plant grown mainly in the cool northern climate of the western Canadian prairies and northern United States. The seed has been grown and cultivated since the times of Babylon. As early as 650 BC, Hippocrates wrote about using flax for the relief of abdominal pains. A little later, Theophrastus recommended the use of flax mucilage as a cough remedy.

Culinary profile

Whole flax seeds are small and reddish brown and impart very little additional flavor when added to foods. However, they can take on a pleasant nutty flavor when roasted.

Cooking with flax

Flax is available as

- oil
- whole seeds
- ground seeds, also known as milled flax or flaxseed meal

You may add flax oil to fruit smoothies or soups. However, flax oil is not recommended for frying. Its high concentration of polyunsaturated fatty acids is very unstable at high temperatures. Whole seeds may be added to granola or used on top of muffins and in breads, hot cereals, rice dishes, or salads. Flax seeds can replace the oil or shortening in a recipe because of their high oil content. If a recipe calls for $1/3$ cup (75 mL) oil, use 1 cup (250 mL) ground flax seeds to replace the oil: a 3:1 substitution ratio. When flax is used instead of oil, baked goods tend to brown more rapidly.

When adding ground flax seeds to a recipe, extra liquid must be added (for every 3 tbsp/45 mL flax, add 1 tbsp/15 mL liquid).

Storing flax

Whole flax seeds that are clean, dry, and of good quality can be stored at room temperature for up to a year. For optimum freshness, flax seeds should be ground as needed. Refrigerate ground flax seeds in an airtight opaque container.

Nutritional profile

Flax offers a wide range of nutritional benefits: a high content of omega-3 fatty acids, particularly alpha-linoleic acid, lignan, and dietary fiber. The nutrient composition of flax also includes a number of important essential minerals. For example, 1 tablespoon (15 mL) of ground flax seeds contains the same amount of magnesium as a banana (34 mg) and the same amount of potassium as a slice of toasted pumpernickel bread (66 mg). It also provides a good source of vitamin E, a potent antioxidant.

Nutritional profile

Ground flax seeds, 3/4 cup (100 g)	Values	% of Daily Value
Calories (kcal)	450	—
Fat (g)	42.0	64.0
Protein (g)	21.0	42.0
Carbohydrates (g)	34.0	11.0
Fiber (g)	28.0	112.0
Vitamin B_1 – thiamin (mg)	0.7	47.0
Vitamin B_2 – riboflavin (mg)	0.3	18.0
Vitamin B_3 – niacin (mg)	4.4	22.0
Vitamin B_6 (mg)	0.8	40.0
Calcium (mg)	250.0	25.0
Iron (mg)	10.0	55.6
Copper (mg)	0.7	35.0
Magnesium (mg)	350.0	87.5
Manganese (mg)	7.0	350.0
Phosphorus (mg)	650.0	65.0
		(Source: Food Processor SQL 2009 edition)

Indian rice grass (Montina)

As its name suggests, Indian rice grass was traditionally eaten by some Native American peoples and used as a reserve food source or ground into flour. The plant is a perennial grass that grows wild in North America, from southern Manitoba to higher elevations in southern California. The grass is very tolerant of drought. The seeds, which resemble millet, are small, round, and dark in color and are covered with white hairs.

Currently, Indian rice grass is grown under the brand name Montina throughout the United States. It is milled, processed, and packaged in a dedicated gluten-free facility in Montana. It is also regularly tested for gluten with the ELISA test before entering the production facility.

Culinary profile

Montina flour has a sweet, nutty, almost wheat-like flavor and texture. It can replace part of the flour used in regular gluten-free baking to improve the fiber and flavor of your baked goods, as well as to enhance the baking performance.

Cooking with Indian rice grass

Indian rice grass flour, manufactured under the brand name Montina Baking Supplement, may be used as a substitute for $\frac{1}{2}$ cup of the amount of rice flour called for in any baking recipe. Amazing Grains Inc. also produces Montina Baking Flour blend, which combines white rice flour, tapioca flour and Indian rice grass. It can be used for a cup-for-cup exchange with any flour.

Storing Indian rice grass

You may store Indian rice grass in a cool, dry location for up to 1 year. Freezing or refrigeration is not required but is advisable if storing for a longer period of time.

Nutritional profile

Indian rice grass is an excellent source of iron and fiber and a source of calcium.

Nutritional profile		
Indian rice grass, $\frac{2}{3}$ cup (100 g)	Values	% of Daily Value
Calories (kcal)	380	—
Fat (g)	3.0	4.6
Protein (g)	17.0	34.0
Carbohydrates (g)	70.0	23.0
Fiber (g)	24.0	96.0
Calcium (mg)	80.0	8.0
Iron (mg)	7.2	40.0
		(Source: www.amazinggrains.com)

Job's tears (hato mugi)

Weed to some, necklace to others, staff of life to others, Job's tears is a very useful and productive grass increasingly viewed as a potential energy source and in some cultures used for its medicinal properties. The grain takes its name from its hard casing, which resembles tear-shaped beads. Before maize became popular in South Asia, Job's tears was rather widely cultivated as a cereal in India. Still regarded as a minor cereal, it is pounded, threshed, and winnowed for use as a cereal or breadstuff. The pounded flour is sometimes mixed with water, like barley for barley water.

The pounded kernel is also made into a sweet dish by frying and coating with sugar. It is also husked and eaten as a snack like peanuts. Beers and wines are made from the fermented grain, and in Korea and China, hato mugi is often made into a tea-like beverage or distilled into liquor. While it may not be found in regular grocery stores across North America, it can be purchased by mail order and is sometimes found in natural food stores.

Culinary profile

Job's tears has a distinctive nutty taste and chewy texture. As in Asian cultures, it may be added to soups and broths. It may also be combined with brown rice or as part of rice mixes to make a tasty side dish in a 1:3 ratio (1 part Job's tears to 3 parts rice).

Cooking with Job's tears

One cup (250 mL) of whole-grain Job's tears will cook in approximately 1 hour when added to boiling water or gluten-free vegetable or chicken stock in a ratio of 1 part grain to 2 parts liquid, to yield $2\frac{1}{2}$ cups (625 mL). Allow the mix to return to a boil and then lower the heat and simmer until the grains swell and become tender.

Job's tears, 1 cup (250 mL)	Liquid	Cooking Time	Yield
Whole grains, uncooked	2 cups (500 mL)	1 hour	$2\frac{1}{2}$ cups (625 mL)

Storing Job's tears

The grain can be stored for several months in the refrigerator if it is sealed in an airtight container, or it can be stored for 6 months or more if kept in the freezer.

Nutritional profile

Job's tears packs a powerful nutrition punch, providing an excellent source of iron — 94% of the daily recommended intake per $3\frac{1}{2}$-ounce (100 gram) serving! It is also an excellent source of bone-strengthening phosphorus and a source of calcium. Definitely worth the effort to obtain it!

Nutritional profile		
Job's tears, whole seed, $2/3$ cup (100 g)	Values	% of Daily Value
Calories (kcal)	372	—
Fat (g)	2.5	4.0
Protein (g)	13.1	26.0
Carbohydrates (g)	72.9	24.0
Fiber (g)	0.8	3.2
Vitamin B_1 – thiamin (mg)	0.44	29.0
Vitamin B_3 – niacin (mg)	2.6	13.0
Calcium (mg)	63.0	6.3
Iron (mg)	16.9	94.0
Phosphorus (mg)	280.0	28.0
		(Source: Food Processor SQL 2009 edition)

Millet

Millet may well be one of the most ancient crops, predating rice and wheat in parts of Asia, India, and Africa. In fact, storage pits, along with the remains of pit houses, pottery, and stone tools related to millet cultivation, have been found in China dating as far back as 8300 BC. In Europe, millet, not corn, was an original ingredient of polenta in Italian cuisine and continues to be used in Russian cuisine as the main ingredient of sweet millet porridge.

Culinary profile

There are several species of millet, of which the most widely cultivated are

- pearl millet
- foxtail millet
- proso millet
- finger millet

The most common variety found in North America is pearl millet, which has a light gold color and resembles mustard seeds in appearance; it brings a sweet, nutty flavor to most meals. Millet grains may be used to make hot breakfast porridge or as a tasty side dish replacing rice or potatoes. It can also make soups and stews hearty and wholesome.

Cooking with millet

Millet may be used as whole grain but is also available as puffed millet or millet flour. Before cooking, rinse millet thoroughly under running water to remove any dirt or debris. To cook, add 1 part millet to $2\frac{1}{2}$ parts boiling water or broth. After the liquid has returned to a boil, turn down the heat, cover, and simmer for about 25 minutes. Fluff with a fork before serving. If you want the millet to have a creamier consistency, stir it frequently, adding a little water until you reach the desired consistency. To impart a nuttier flavor, you may choose to toast millet in a dry skillet over medium heat, stirring constantly until fragrant, for about 5 minutes.

Millet, 1 cup (250 mL)	Liquid	Cooking Time	Yield	Additional Info
Whole grain, uncooked	$2\frac{1}{2}$ cups (625 mL)	25 minutes	2 cups (500 mL)	Toast millet for 6 minutes to bring out its delicious nutty flavor.

Storing millet

Millet may be available prepackaged in bags or in bulk containers. Millet is prone to becoming rancid quickly because of its high content of polyunsaturated fatty acids. If stored in a cool, dry, dark place it can keep for several months.

Nutritional profile

Millet, cooked, $\frac{2}{3}$ cup (100 g)	Values	% of Daily Value
Calories (kcal)	119	—
Fat (g)	1.0	1.5
Protein (g)	3.5	7.2
Carbohydrates (g)	23.7	7.9
Fiber (g)	1.3	5.2
Vitamin B_1 – thiamin (mg)	0.1	7.0
Vitamin B_3 – niacin (mg)	1.33	6.7
Vitamin B_6 (mg)	0.1	1.4
Folate (mcg)	19.0	4.8
Copper (mg)	0.16	8.0
Iron (mg)	0.63	3.5.0
Magnesium (mg)	44.0	11.0
Manganese (mg)	0.3	13.6
Phosphorus (mg)	100.0	10.0
(Source: Food Processor SQL 2009 edition)		

Potato starch and potato flour

Potatoes are the fourth-largest crop in the world, behind wheat, rice, and corn.

Culinary profile

Potato flour is made from the whole potato, including the skin. It is darker and heavier than potato starch and has a definite potato flavor. Potato starch is made from the starchy portion of the potato; it is less expensive and lower on the nutritional scale and has no discernible flavor.

Cooking with potato starch and potato flour

Potato flour is often added to gluten-free baking mixes for breads and pastries, as it retains moisture well. At home, potato starch is a good wheat flour substitute when frying foods in oil. Its bland taste lends itself well to thickening sauces and gravies.

Storing potato starch

Store in the refrigerator or the freezer.

Nutritional profile		
Potato flour, ⅔ cup (100 g)	Values	% of Daily Value
Calories (kcal)	357	—
Fat (g)	0.34	0.5
Protein (g)	7.0	13.8
Carbohydrates (g)	83.0	27.7
Fiber (g)	6.0	23.6
Vitamin B_1 – thiamin (mg)	0.2	15.2
Vitamin B_3 – niacin (mg)	3.5	17.5
Vitamin B_6 (mg)	0.8	34.5
Magnesium (mg)	65.0	16.3
Manganese (mg)	0.3	16.0
Phosphorus (mg)	168.0	16.8
Potassium (mg)	1001.0	28.6
(Source: Food Processor SQL 2009 edition)		

Oats

Until recently, oats were out of bounds for those with celiac disease, mostly because of concerns about cross-contamination from gluten-containing grains such as wheat or barley during harvesting or processing. Happily, this has changed and most celiac research centers, support groups, and other organizations in North America and around the world recognize that small amounts of pure, uncontaminated oats may be tolerated by most (but not all) individuals with celiac disease. There are now several suppliers of pure, uncontaminated oats throughout North America: Cream Hill Estates of Quebec, Canada; Only Oats of Saskatchewan, Canada; and Gluten Free Oats of Wyoming, USA. These companies grow, harvest, and process oats that are thoroughly tested at every critical stage:

- as seed
- at planting
- while growing in the field
- at harvesting
- during transport
- in storage
- during processing and packaging

Culinary profile

Oats owe their distinctive flavor and texture to the roasting process that they undergo after harvesting and cleaning. Pure, uncontaminated oats come in several forms:

- **Groats** are unflattened kernels made in the original Scottish tradition. They have a sweet, nutty taste and may be used as breakfast cereal or for stuffing.

- **Rolled oats** are what people refer to as "oatmeal." Their flat shape is the result of steaming the groats and then passing them through smooth, then corrugated rollers that render them into different thicknesses (regular, medium, or thick rolled oats). Rolled oats have a chewy texture and complement many types of meals while being very filling and satisfying.

- **Oat flour** is made from finely ground groats, which contain much of the bran, making the flour just as nutritious as the grain itself. Just like the groats, oat flour has a sweet, nutty flavor.

Cooking with oats

Oats, 1 cup (250 mL)	Liquid	Cooking Time	Yield	Additional Info
Groats, uncooked	3 cups (750 mL)	45 minutes	2 cups (500 mL)	
Rolled oats	2¼ cups (550 mL)	5–15 minutes	2 cups (500 mL)	Soaking oats for 15 minutes reduces cooking time by half.

Storing oats

It is generally recommended that oats be purchased in small quantities since the grain has a high content of polyunsaturated fats and risks becoming rancid. Oatmeal should be stored in a tightly lidded container in a cool, dry place for up to 2 months. Manufacturers of pure, uncontaminated oats have slightly differing recommendations for storing oats:

Gluten-Free Oats: Keep products refrigerated.
Cream Hill Estates: No refrigeration needed. Store in a cool, dry place.
Only Oats: No refrigeration needed. Store in a cool, dry place.

Nutritional profile

Oats are a very good source of selenium. Like vitamin E, this trace mineral acts as part of the antioxidant enzyme glutathione peroxidase and has its own antioxidant activity, which helps strengthen the immune system.

Nutritional profile

Oats, rolled, dry, ¼ cup (39 g)	Values	% of Daily Value
Calories (kcal)	152	—
Fat (g)	2.5	3.9
Protein (g)	6.2	12.5
Carbohydrates (g)	26.0	8.7
Fiber (g)	4.1	16.5
Vitamin B_1 – thiamin (mg)	0.2	14.0
Iron (mg)	1.6	9.0
Magnesium (mg)	57.7	14.0
Manganese (mg)	1.4	70.8
Phosphorus (mg)	185.0	18.5
Selenium (mcg)	13.3	19.0
Zinc (mg)	1.2	8.0

(Source: Food Processor SQL 2009 edition)

Quinoa

"The gold of the Incas," as it used to be known in the Andean region of South America, quinoa is a grain being rediscovered in North America for its versatility and nutritional benefits. We see quinoa being used more often in recipes as a natural alternative to couscous and rice. Quinoa is actually a seed, from a plant closely related to beets, spinach, and tumbleweed. Most of the quinoa available in North America is grown in the Andean country of Bolivia, where it thrives at very high altitudes.

Culinary profile

Quinoa resembles millet in shape but comes in various colored varieties, such as yellow, red, and sometimes black. The most common complaint about quinoa refers to its bitter taste. Quinoa grains are naturally coated with saponin, a natural detergent through which the plant protects itself against birds and insects. However, most distributors of quinoa seeds have processes in place to remove this coating. Still, it may also be a good idea for you to rinse the grain before using. Quinoa flour, ground from whole seeds, has a delicate, nutty flavor.

Cooking with quinoa

Quinoa may be found in a variety of forms:

- whole grains
- flour
- flakes
- pasta

Whole-grain quinoa cooks relatively fast — in about 15 minutes when cooked in boiling water or broth at a ratio of 1:2 (1 part quinoa to 2 parts liquid). You will know quinoa is ready to serve when you see the seed break through its casing and a white line appear around the outside. Remove from heat and let stand, covered, for 5 minutes.

The seeds may also be cooked in the microwave on High for 12 minutes using the same ratio as mentioned above. You may want to stir it once midway through before returning it to the oven to complete cooking.

In baking, 1/4 cup (60 mL) quinoa flour may be substituted for rice flour to add a nutritional punch to your muffins or flatbreads. Quinoa flour has a very strong, nutty flavor that can sometimes overpower baking recipes. Quinoa flakes make an excellent hot breakfast cereal. Quinoa flour can also be combined with other gluten-free flours and brans, such as corn or rice, to make pasta. To cook quinoa pasta, bring water to a boil. Mix 1 part quinoa pasta into 2 parts boiling water and stir occasionally for 13 to 15 minutes. Remove from heat and drain.

Quinoa, 1 cup (250 mL)	Liquid	Cooking Time	Yield	Additional Info
Whole grain, uncooked	2 cups (500 mL)	15 minutes	3–4 cups (750 mL–1 L)	
Flakes, breakfast cereal	3 cups (750 mL)	1.5–2 minutes	3 cups (750 mL)	You may prepare flakes in the microwave; cook on High for 6½ minutes for 4 servings.
Pasta, uncooked	2½ cups (625 mL)	15 minutes	1½ cups (375 mL)	

Storing quinoa

Whole-grain quinoa is best kept in an airtight container in the refrigerator for up to 6 months. Flour is best stored in the freezer. Quinoa is relatively high in polyunsaturated fats, so you need to ensure that the package you are buying is fresh; choose to buy from a source that has high turnover. Ensure that the packaging has no evidence of moisture.

Nutritional profile

Quinoa is a very good source of manganese and a good source of magnesium, iron, copper, and phosphorus. It is also a complete protein.

Nutritional profile

Quinoa, cooked, ½ cup (100 g)	Values	% of Daily Value
Calories (kcal)	120	—
Fat (g)	1.9	3.0
Protein (g)	4.4	9.0
Carbohydrates (g)	21.0	7.0
Fiber (g)	3.0	11.0
Folate (mcg)	42.0	10.5
Iron (mg)	1.5	8.0
Magnesium (mg)	64.0	16.0
Manganese (mg)	0.63	62.0
Phosphorus (mg)	152.0	15.0
Copper (mg)	0.19	10.0
		(Source: Food Processor SQL 2009 edition)

Rice

One of the most popular cereal grains, rice supplies almost half the daily calories of almost half of the world's population, especially in China, Japan, India, Bangladesh, Cambodia, Indonesia, Laos, Thailand, and Vietnam. Although it has a low protein content compared to other grains, brown rice ranks higher than wheat for available carbohydrates and digestible energy.

Culinary profile

Most whole-grain rice is brown, although specialty varieties such as black, red, and japonica are quickly becoming popular, especially in the form of rice mixes. The harvested rice kernel, known as paddy, or rough, rice, is enclosed by the hull, or husk. Milling usually removes both the hull and bran layers of the kernel, and a coating of glucose and talc is sometimes applied to give the kernel a glossy finish. Rice that is processed to remove only the husks, called brown rice, contains about 8% protein and small amounts of fats; it is a source of thiamin, niacin, riboflavin, iron, and calcium. The bran remaining in whole-grain brown rice contains important phytonutrients thought to reduce the risk of heart attacks, certain cancers, and type 2 diabetes and to aid in weight control. Rice that is milled to remove the bran as well is called white rice.

Cooking with rice

Rice is classified by the size of its grain:

- *Long-grain rice* is slender, meaning that the grains separate while cooking, giving you an "al dente" quality suitable for side dishes or as a bed for sauces.
- *Medium-grain rice* is shorter and plumper, making it a good candidate for paella or risotto.
- *Short-grain rice* is round, with moist grains that stick together when cooked.

Other specialty varieties of rice include

- **Glutinous rice**, also referred to as "sticky rice," is used for sushi and rice balls. Do not be concerned by the word *glutinous*— this rice is also gluten-free.
- **Basmati rice** is an aromatic long-grain rice grown in the foothills of the Himalayas and is especially popular in India. The cooked grains are dry and fluffy, so they make a nice bed for curries and sauces. Basmati is available as either white or brown rice. Brown basmati has more fiber and a stronger flavor, but it takes twice as long to cook.

- **Black rice**, including black japonica rice, Chinese black rice, Thai black sticky rice, and Indonesian black rice, is high in fiber and has a strong, nutty taste. Black rice has a deep black color that turns dark purple when cooked, which suggests the presence of phytonutrients: important antioxidants involved in reducing the risk of heart disease and several cancers and promoting overall health. It also provides a relatively high content of iron.

- **Red rice**, such as Buthanese red rice, Himalayan red rice, and Camargue red rice, has a strong, nutty flavor and cooks faster than brown rice. Its rich red color suggests the presence of phytonutrients, a source of heart-healthy antioxidants. You may substitute this rice with a North American equivalent derived from basmati rice, called wehani.

- **Rice flour** (white or brown) is a very popular flour substitute in gluten-free baking. Because it contains volatile oils, it is quite perishable. Store brown rice flour in the refrigerator for up to 5 months or in the freezer for up to 1 year.

Cooking rice

Rice, 1 cup (250 mL)	Liquid	Cooking Time	Yield	Additional Info
Whole-grain rice, uncooked	2½ cups (625 mL)	45–50 minutes	3 cups (750 mL)	
Glutinous rice, uncooked	1 cup (250 mL)	20 minutes	2 cups (500 mL)	For best results, this type of rice requires a rice steamer.
Basmati rice, uncooked	1½ cups (375 mL)	20–30 minutes	2½ cups (625 mL)	Do not peek or stir the rice before the approximate cooking time is complete.

Nutritional profile		
Long-grain brown rice, cooked, 1/2 cup (100 g)	**Values**	**% of Daily Value**
Calories (kcal)	111	—
Fat (g)	0.9	1.4
Protein (g)	2.6	5.0
Carbohydrates (g)	23.0	7.7
Fiber (g)	1.8	7.2
Folate (mcg)	43.0	11.0
Manganese (mg)	0.91	45.0
Phosphorus (mg)	83.0	8.3
Selenium (mcg)	9.8	14.0
	(Source: Food Processor SQL 2009 edition)	

Sorghum

Also known as milo, sorghum is a tropical plant, one of the most important crops in Africa, Asia, and Latin America. It has a very high nutritional value as a powerful source of antioxidants and works very well in gluten-free baking recipes. Sorghum may be used to make tortillas (Latin America), a thin porridge known as *bouille* in Africa and Asia, couscous in Africa, *injera* in Ethiopia, or *bhakri*, an unleavened bread that is a staple in India. In North America, sorghum is also used to make gluten-free beer.

Tortilla chips may be made by mixing sorghum with maize and cassava.

Culinary profile

Whole-grain sorghum has a mild taste that becomes stronger with toasting. Sorghum flour is bland and works as a very good replacement for wheat flour in most baking recipes. It may be a component of a gluten-free flour mix or may be used as the sole flour in puddings, pancakes, crêpes, tortillas, or banana breads.

Cooking with sorghum

It is best to soak whole-grain sorghum overnight in water. To cook on the stovetop, add 1 cup (250 mL) sorghum grains to 2 cups (500 mL) boiling water. Reduce heat and let simmer, covered, for 50 minutes. Remove from heat and let stand for 10 minutes. Puffed sorghum may be used to make granola cereals or dry snacks and may be added to soups instead of other grains. Sorghum flour makes a great addition to recipes for pizza dough, pie crust, waffles, and pancakes.

Sorghum, 1 cup (250 mL)	Liquid	Cooking Time	Yield	Additional Info
Whole grains	2 cups (500 mL)	50–60 minutes	2½ cups (625 mL)	

Storing sorghum

Keep sorghum flour in a tightly lidded container in a cool, dark place for up to 1 month. You can extend the shelf life to 6 months by refrigerating it or up to 1 year by freezing it.

Nutritional profile

Antioxidants, such as phenols and tannins, have the ability to neutralize cellular by-products called free radicals, caused by environmental pollutants, poor nutrition, drugs, smoking, and excessive alcohol consumption. Studies have revealed that specialty varieties of sorghum, such as brown sorghum and sorghum bran, are a surprisingly good source of cancer-fighting antioxidants. Sorghum bran contains more antioxidants than blueberries, strawberries, or plums.

Nutritional profile

Sorghum, uncooked, ½ cup (100 g)	Values	% of Daily Value
Calories (kcal)	339	—
Fat (g)	3.3	5.0
Protein (g)	11.3	22.6
Carbohydrates (g)	74.6	25.0
Fiber (g)	6.3	25.0
Vitamin B_1 – thiamin (mg)	0.24	16.0
Vitamin B_3 – niacin (mg)	2.93	15.0
Iron (mg)	4.4	24.0
Phosphorus (mg)	287.0	28.7
		(Source: Food Processor SQL 2009 edition)

Tapioca

Also known as cassava, yucca, and manioc, tapioca is a tropical tuber grown throughout Brazil. Long and cylinder-like in shape, manioc root has a light brown fibrous skin similar to a potato or yam. The inside is white and starchy. Tapioca has many applications in Southeast Asia, India, and South America, ranging from tapioca "chips" to puddings, porridge, sweet bubble teas, and fish curries.

Culinary profile

Tapioca can be used as a starch or as granules known as pearl tapioca. The starch is a fine white powder with a mildly sweet taste and may be used as an instant thickening powder for soups, gravies, and sauces.

Cooking with tapioca starch

Tapioca starch works very well in gluten-free flour mixes and gives loaves, banana breads, and pancakes a chewy texture. To make tapioca pudding, pearls may be soaked in water overnight. To make drinks, you may boil tapioca pearls for 25 minutes, until they are cooked thoroughly and chewy but not gummy, then allow them to cool. If not used immediately, they may be kept for hours in a syrup of sugar or honey.

Storing tapioca starch

Tapioca starch has a shelf life of approximately 1 year if kept in an airtight container in a dry place. Once opened, tapioca pearls need to be kept tightly sealed to prevent loss of moisture. Store in a cool, dry place for up to 6 months.

Nutritional profile		
Tapioca pearls, dry, ½ cup (76 g)	Values	% of Daily Value
Calories (kcal)	272	—
Fat (g)	0.0	0.0
Protein (g)	0.1	0.3
Carbohydrates (g)	67.0	22
Fiber (g)	0.7	3.0
Folate (mcg)	3.0	0.8
Iron (mg)	1.2	6.7
(Source: Food Processor SQL 2009 edition)		

Teff

Teff (also known as tef) is a grass native to Ethiopia, where it is used to make the country's staple bread, *injera*. It is also widely grown in South Africa, India, Australia, and the northwestern USA. The teff grain is extremely small and ranges in color from milky white to black. While it is less well known in North America, its popularity is on the rise thanks to its stellar nutritional profile and delicious taste — and it is gluten-free.

Culinary profile

Teff is available as whole grains or flour. The lighter grain has a mild, hazelnut-like taste, while brown teff has a molasses-like sweetness to it. Teff flour is made from brown teff and has a slightly strong, nutty flavor with a sweet undertone. Teff flour made from white grain is milder. Teff flour is a great addition to your gluten-free flour baking mixes. It works well in breads, pancakes, waffles, pie crusts, and cookies.

Cooking with teff

Teff grain makes great pilaf, replacing rice or potatoes as a side dish for your meals. It works well when combined with kasha (roasted buckwheat), millet, or brown rice. It can also serve as stuffing or porridge. Because it becomes gelatinous when cooked, teff is particularly well suited to thicken stews, gravies, sauces, and soups.

Teff, ½ cup (125 mL)	Liquid	Cooking Time	Yield	Additional Info
Whole grain, uncooked	1½ cups (375 mL)	20–25 minutes	1 cup (250 mL)	

Storing teff

Cooking experts recommend that teff be stored in containers with tight lids in a cool, dark, dry place for up to 1 month. You may store teff in the refrigerator for up to 6 months or in the freezer for up to 1 year.

Nutritional profile

Among grains, teff is a nutritional powerhouse. It's an excellent source of protein, calcium, iron, zinc, copper, phosphorus, and other important nutrients.

Wild rice

Wild rice is not a grain, as its name may suggest, but a grass that grows extensively in shallow lakes and streams. It is native to the North American continent and has been harvested for centuries by Native people of the northern Midwest and in Manitoba, Saskatchewan, and Minnesota.

Nutritional profile

Teff, dry, 1/2 cup (100 g)	Values	% of Daily Value
Calories (kcal)	367	—
Fat (g)	2.38	3.66
Protein (g)	13.3	26.6
Carbohydrates (g)	73.13	24.0
Fiber (g)	8.0	32.0
Vitamin B_1 – thiamin (mg)	0.39	26.0
Vitamin B_2 – riboflavin (mg)	0.27	16.0
Vitamin B_3 – niacin (mg)	3.36	17.0
Vitamin B_6 (mg)	0.48	26.0
Calcium (mg)	180	18.0
Iron (mg)	0.81	40.5
Copper (mg)	7.63	42.4
Magnesium (mg)	184.0	46.0
Manganese (mg)	9.24	462.0
Phosphorus (mg)	429.0	43.0
Zinc (mg)	3.63	24.0
		(Source: Food Processor SQL 2009 edition)

Culinary profile

Wild rice has a chewy texture and a smoky, nutty flavor that lends itself to game and poultry and gives character to any grain side dish. It is most often consumed in mixtures with other types of rice or grains. It also blends well with strong flavors, such as mushrooms, dried fruits, and nuts, and strongly flavored fruits, such as mango, pomegranate, and cranberries. Wild rice flour is gray-brown to black and has a hearty, unique flavor. It is nutritious and a valuable wheat flour substitute. Wild rice flour can be substituted in some recipes, though results are best when it is mixed with other flours. Add to pancake batter, muffins, scones, and bread and substitute up to 1/3 cup (75 mL) wild rice flour for any other flour you are using, such as white rice flour.

Wild rice, 1 cup (250 mL)	Liquid	Cooking Time	Yield	Additional Info
Whole grain, uncooked	2–3 cups (500–750 mL)	45–50 minutes	3 1/2 cups (875 mL)	Rinse thoroughly before cooking.

Nutritional profile

Wild rice is easily digestible, high in fiber and protein (double that of brown rice), and a source of vitamin B, iron, thiamin, riboflavin, niacin, calcium, phosphorus, and carbohydrate.

Nutritional profile		
Wild rice, cooked, 2/3 cup (100 g)	Values	% of Daily Value
Calories (kcal)	100	—
Fat (g)	0.34	0.5
Protein (g)	3.99	8.0
Carbohydrates (g)	21.0	7.0
Fiber (g)	1.8	7.2
Vitamin B_3 – niacin (mg)	1.3	6.4
Vitamin B_6 (mg)	0.14	6.8
Folate (mcg)	26.0	6.5
Magnesium (mg)	32.0	8.0
Phosphorus (mg)	82.0	8.2
Manganese (mg)	0.28	14.0
Zinc (mg)	1.34	8.9

(Source: Food Processor SQL 2009 edition)

CASE HISTORY
Adapting to a gluten-free diet

While Erin had previous experience with a wheat-free diet, she needed to learn more about specific toxic ingredients that would affect her and to be more scrupulous about cross-contamination in her home. We identified food ingredients that she needed to avoid and foods that potentially contained them. We also met at the grocery store where she frequently shopped and identified foods that she could enjoy without fear of gluten, foods that demanded caution, and foods to avoid. We also looked at alternatives for gluten-containing foods.

Based on her lifestyle and food preferences, we put together a meal plan emphasizing foods and meals that would provide her with much-needed iron. We also took a look at good sources of calcium in her diet, since she still experienced lactose intolerance and her bone mass may have been affected by many years of malabsorption.

A few months later, Erin's iron levels were on the rise. She had identified ways to eliminate cross-contamination in the home. Her challenge remained eating out with friends. We looked at her favorite cuisines and restaurants and identified menu items that could be ordered specifically gluten-free, discussing strategies to communicate with restaurant chefs about her needs. This was difficult for her. As a young adult she found it hard to speak up about her needs, especially when they interfered with her social life. To make that job easier, I suggested that Erin contact the restaurant or bar ahead of time to inquire about alternatives and speak to the chef. It took a bit of preplanning on her part, but it worked. And she found that her friends were very supportive!

Part 3

Maintaining Good Nutrition

Maintaining Good Nutrition

While gluten-free foods are becoming more common in the marketplace, they are typically not fortified, leading to nutrient deficiencies, and provide higher calories and fat, leading to weight gain for those who depend on them. People with celiac disease eating a gluten-free diet may simply become undernourished and overfed. To counter these tendencies, you may need to supplement your diet with specific nutrients and monitor your energy balance.

Essential Nutrients

Despite consuming healthy gluten-free grains, fresh fruits, vegetables, and protein sources, individuals with celiac disease continue to be challenged by nutrient deficiencies that compromise their health and well-being. A recent study revealed that a significant percentage of participants with celiac disease did not get their recommended daily intake of many essential nutrients:

- vitamin B_1 (thiamin): 58.7%
- vitamin B_2 (riboflavin): 24.8%
- vitamin B_3 (niacin): 29.4%
- vitamin B_6: 34.9%
- vitamin B_{12}: 29.4%
- folate: 85.3%
- vitamin D: 92.7%
- iron: 41.3%
- calcium: 81.7%
- fiber: 74.3%

These deficiencies can cause serious illness. For example, fiber deficiency leads to constipation and gastrointestinal discomfort, calcium and vitamin D deficiencies lead to bone loss through osteopenia and osteoporosis, while iron deficiency anemia leads to a weak immune system and fatigue.

Food basics

About 40 nutrients are known to be essential to human beings to maintain life, foster growth, and repair tissues. Food provides us with nutrients the body cannot make at all or those the body makes only in insufficient quantities, such as vitamin D. These are *essential* because they are absolutely needed to meet physiological requirements. Our diet supplies these essential nutrients, but sometimes nutrient supplements are needed.

Most foods contain mixtures of macronutrients (that provide us with energy) and micronutrients (that enable metabolism of macronutrients).

Macronutrients	Micronutrients
• Carbohydrate • Fat • Protein	• Vitamins • Minerals • Amino acids • Essential fatty acids • Enzymes

Did You Know?
Power snack

Gluten-free protein bars are usually fortified with vitamins and minerals, and they make a great convenient and portable snack when you are on the go.

Energy

The body uses carbohydrates, fat, and protein to fuel its metabolic and physical activities. The energy used to keep the heart beating, the brain thinking, and the legs running comes from these compounds. If the body has an excess of any of the three energy-yielding nutrients, it rearranges them into storage compounds, mostly as fat, to be drawn upon between meals and overnight. This is why, if you take in more energy than you expend, you gain weight as body fat.

Vitamins

Vitamins help the body convert macronutrients into useable energy. They assist other nutrients to digest, absorb, and metabolize food. One vitamin enables your eyes to see in the dark; another helps to protect the lungs from air pollution. It takes sometimes two or three vitamins acting together to help the bones get stronger or to replace old red blood cells with new ones. Every action in the body requires the assistance of vitamins.

Did You Know?
Fiber functions

The fibers are a class of compounds related to the carbohydrate group. Unlike the carbohydrates, however, fibers pass through the body mostly undigested, yielding little or no energy. Fibers keep the digestive tract muscles healthy and strong and also carry harmful substances out of the body, helping to prevent heart disease and cancer.

Cooking tips to help preserve vitamins

Because of their organic and complex nature, vitamins are vulnerable to being altered and losing their potency when exposed to heat, light and chemical agents. Here are some tips for saving vitamin potency while cooking foods.

• Use small amounts of water when boiling foods.
• Shorten the cooking time of fruits and vegetables as much as possible.
• Choose steaming, blanching, or poaching more often.

Minerals

Minerals play an essential role in the body's chemistry, ranging from being the main components in bones and teeth to influencing the chemistry of bodily fluids. Their concentration is typically measured in micrograms or milligrams. Minerals are indestructible and do not require special handling the way vitamins do — in other words, they are not affected by heat, light, or exposure to air. They can, however, be bound by substances that make it hard for the body to absorb them.

Water

Water is often taken for granted, but it forms a major part of almost every body tissue. By supplying a medium for transportation of vital nutrients to cells and carrying waste away from them, it provides the environment in which nearly all of the body's metabolic activities take place. Water is found in nearly all types of foods, from fruits and vegetables to meats, fish, poultry, grains, and legumes.

Nutrient Deficiencies in Celiac Disease

In celiac disease, the damage to the intestinal lining affects the absorption of several vitamins and minerals that are essential to health and well-being. Different parts of the small intestine that sustain the damage are responsible for the absorption of different types of nutrients.

Duodenum and jejunum absorb
- protein
- sugars (including lactose, the principal sugar in milk)
- iron
- calcium
- zinc
- folate
- fat-soluble vitamins (K, A, D, and E)

Ileum absorbs
- vitamin B_{12}

Poor nutritional status affects immunity and the ability to prevent complications of malabsorption typical of celiac disease: lactose intolerance, calcium deficiency leading to osteopenia or osteoporosis, vitamin D deficiency, iron deficiency anemia, and folate and vitamin B_{12} deficiency. Remember that these deficiencies can be corrected by following the gluten-free diet for life.

Lactose intolerance

Lactose intolerance is the condition that results from the body's inability to break down and absorb the milk sugar called lactose. Lactose is a disaccharide, meaning it is a larger sugar made up of two smaller sugars called monosaccharides. The agent responsible for splitting lactose into its individual components and making them available for absorption into the body is the enzyme *lactase*, which resides in the microvilli of intestinal cells.

When lactose cannot be properly broken down into its individual components, it remains in the intestine undigested, attracting water and causing bloating, abdominal discomfort, and diarrhea — the main symptoms of lactose intolerance. The lactose also becomes food for intestinal bacteria residing in the colon, which multiply and produce irritating acid and gas, further contributing to the discomfort and diarrhea. Symptoms typically occur 30 minutes to 2 hours after consuming milk, other dairy products, or meals prepared with these ingredients.

Lactase deficiency

When lactose intolerance develops, three causes are usually explored:

1. **Primary lactase deficiency.** This is the most common cause of lactase deficiency, affecting as many as 75% of adults throughout the world. As we age there is a natural decline in the amount of lactase enzyme available to break down lactose, causing decreased tolerance of dairy products. This natural decline is genetically determined and occurs at different rates in different ethnic groups. The frequency of primary lactase deficiency can range from as little as 5% in Scandinavian and northern European populations to up to 90% in groups of African, Jewish, and Asian descent. In North American adults, the prevalence rate follows a similar pattern depending on ethnic origin.

2. **Secondary lactase deficiency.** This is usually environmentally induced and temporary in nature, meaning that individuals can usually recover and slowly regain the ability to tolerate milk and dairy products. This type of lactase deficiency results from injury to the small intestine caused by certain types of medical treatments, such as chemotherapy, or it may occur because of gastrointestinal infections or inflammatory bowel disease, such as Crohn's disease. Celiac disease is another cause of secondary lactase deficiency. Once the disease or injury resolves, lactase reappears on the surface of the intestinal mucosa and proper lactose digestion resumes.

3. **Congenital lactase deficiency.** This type of lactase deficiency occurs because of a congenital absence (absence from birth) of lactase due to a mutation in the gene that is responsible for producing it. This is a very rare but severe type of lactose intolerance, and the symptoms begin shortly after birth.

Did You Know?
Genetic reversal

The rate of lactose intolerance in African Americans has fallen from 100% to 75% because of interracial reproduction. Similarly, Native Americans have shown a steady rise in their ability to digest lactose as their gene pool has blended with that of other North Americans.

Testing for lactose intolerance

Diagnosing lactose intolerance from symptoms alone can be difficult because, just as in celiac disease, they are not specific to this condition alone. You may experience bloating, gas, and diarrhea from irritable bowel syndrome, a flare-up of ulcerative colitis, or Crohn's disease. It is important to use a formal method of testing and to confirm your diagnosis with a physician.

Hydrogen breath test

During this test you will be asked to drink a lactose-loaded beverage. If you are lacking sufficient amounts of lactase enzymes, the undigested lactose will be fermented by colonic bacteria and hydrogen gas will result. The total amount of lactose you consume is very important — if you are only slightly intolerant to lactose, an amount of 10 to 12 grams of lactose (equivalent to $\frac{1}{2}$ cup/125 mL milk) may not create symptoms and your intolerance may well go undiagnosed. However, an amount of 50 grams of lactose (equivalent to 1 quart/1 L of milk) will be more relevant to your case.

Stool acidity test

This test is used for infants and children to measure the amount of acid in the stool.

Dietary management of lactose intolerance

There is a large variation in the degree of lactose intolerance among people. For those with primary lactase deficiency, tolerance can range from as little as a couple of tablespoons (30 mL) of yogurt to up to $\frac{1}{2}$ cup (125 mL) of white milk. However, most can improve their tolerance to milk and dairy products by slowly and very gradually incorporating them in small amounts into their diet. This improvement happens because the gastrointestinal bacteria are able to adapt to the lactose load without causing symptoms.

Those with secondary lactose intolerance resulting from celiac disease may need to temporarily eliminate lactose until the villi of the small intestine are healed and the levels of lactase enzyme are restored. This may take a few weeks to months, depending on the individual response to the gluten-free diet.

Food labels

While lactose is not listed on the Nutrition Facts label, you may still be able to check how much lactose is present in specific foods. Take, for example, hard aged or semi-soft cheese. The Nutrition Facts table lists "Carbohydrates," and further down, as a subheading, you will see the term "Sugars." Because natural cheeses do not have added sweeteners, the amount listed under Sugars refers solely to the amount of lactose in that product.

Low-lactose dairy products

The following dairy products contain very little lactose and may be easier to start incorporating into your diet. Each food has been rated on the lactose-free scale.

Lactose-free scale

Level 1: Foods contain very small amounts or traces of lactose, making them easy to incorporate in a gluten-free and lactose-free diet.

Level 2: Foods contain small amounts of lactose and can be gradually introduced in small amounts into your diet as you check your tolerance for them.

Food	Serving Size	Amount of Lactose	Lactose-free Scale (see above)
Butter	1 tsp (5 mL)	Trace	Level 1
Blue cheese	1 oz (30 g)	1 g	Level 1
Brick	1 oz (30 g)	1 g	Level 1
Brie	1 oz (30 g)	< 1 g	Level 1
Camembert	1 oz (30 g)	< 1 g	Level 1
Cheddar	1 oz (30 g)	< 1 g	Level 1
Edam	1 oz (30 g)	< 1 g	Level 1
Gouda	1 oz (30 g)	< 1 g	Level 1
Gruyère	1 oz (30 g)	< 1 g	Level 1
Gorgonzola	1 oz (30 g)	< 1 g	Level 1
Lappi	1 oz (30 g)	0 g	Level 1
Liedenkranz	1 oz (30 g)	< 1 g	Level 1
Mozzarella, full-fat milk	1 oz (30 g)	1 g	Level 1
Mozzarella, part-skim	1 oz (30 g)	1 g	Level 1
Muenster	1 oz (30 g)	< 1 g	Level 1
Parmesan	1 oz (30 g)	1 g	Level 1
Provolone	1 oz (30 g)	1 g	Level 1
Romano	1 oz (30 g)	1 g	Level 1
Swiss	1 oz (30 g)	1 g	Level 1
Processed cheese	1 oz (30 g)	1 g	Level 1
Lactose-free milk	1 cup (250 mL)	1 g	Level 1
Cream cheese	2 tbsp (30 mL)	2 g	Level 2
American cheese spread	2 tbsp (30 mL)	2 g	Level 2
Coffee whitener	1 tbsp (15 mL)	2 g	Level 2
Yogurt, plain, 90% lactose-free	$\frac{1}{2}$ cup (125 mL)	4 g	Level 2

Nutrient supplements for managing lactose intolerance

Over-the-counter lactase enzyme supplements are available in tablet or liquid form. Their role is to supplement the lactase enzymes produced by your own intestine and to help break down lactose in milk products or meals that may contain milk or milk products.

Calcium caution

When people learn they are lactose intolerant, they typically react by reducing or even eliminating milk and dairy products, which can result in a calcium deficiency. In this circumstance, it is extremely important to find other sources of calcium.

Did You Know?
Cocoa treats

Pure cocoa powder is lactose-free, fat-free, and chock full of antioxidants. If you are lactose intolerant, you may enjoy it with lactose-free milk or non-dairy milks such as soy, rice, almond, or potato milk. High-quality dark chocolate made from cocoa butter, cocoa liquor, lecithin, and sugar is both lactose-free and gluten-free.

Recommended calcium intake by age group	
Age Group	Dietary Reference Intakes (mg/day)
0–6 months	210
7–12 months	270
1–3 years	500
4–8 years	800
9–18 years (women)	1,300
9–18 years (men)	1,300
19–50 years (women)	1,000
19–50 years (men)	1,000
51+ years (men and women)	1,200
Pregnancy, 14–18 years	1,300
Pregnancy, 19–50 years	1,000
Lactation, 14–18 years	1,300
Lactation, 19–50 years	1,000

(*Source:* Adapted from National Academy of Sciences, Institute of Medicine, *Dietary Reference Intakes*, 2004.)

Food sources of calcium

Fortunately, many foods, dairy and non-dairy, can provide adequate intake of calcium. To meet the recommendations, take into account your overall daily intake of calcium. The bar graph on page 101 ranks the calcium content in foods from richest to poorest.

Osteopenia and osteoporosis

Our bones are assumed to be static, much like bricks in the foundation of a house. However, they are living organisms, constantly building and breaking up again. The bones are strongest and most dense in young adulthood. Up to about the age of 30, bone-building activities are dominant. For a while after, the bones stop growing and a balance dominates in which bone building and bone breakdown happen at similar rates. As the years pass, bone dismantling dominates, resulting in loss of bone mass.

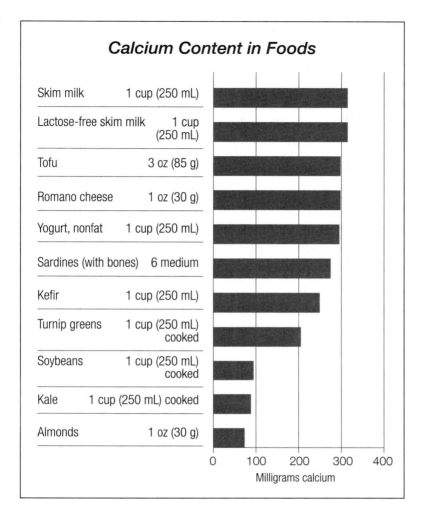

Calcium Content in Foods

Food	Serving
Skim milk	1 cup (250 mL)
Lactose-free skim milk	1 cup (250 mL)
Tofu	3 oz (85 g)
Romano cheese	1 oz (30 g)
Yogurt, nonfat	1 cup (250 mL)
Sardines (with bones)	6 medium
Kefir	1 cup (250 mL)
Turnip greens	1 cup (250 mL) cooked
Soybeans	1 cup (250 mL) cooked
Kale	1 cup (250 mL) cooked
Almonds	1 oz (30 g)

Milligrams calcium (0, 100, 200, 300, 400)

Bones are made of minerals, including calcium, phosphorus, and magnesium. Calcium is the predominant mineral, accounting for 80% of bone chemistry. Many factors affect calcium absorption, but on average, adults absorb about 30% of the calcium they ingest. The stomach's acidity favors calcium absorption by helping to keep it soluble. Vitamin D helps to make the necessary calcium-binding protein in the absorptive cells of the GI tract. Other factors also contribute to maintaining bone health, including vitamin K, protein, potassium, and magnesium.

Celiac disease and bone deterioration

When celiac disease goes undiagnosed for a long period of time, the damage to the lining in the small intestine — where the bulk of mineral absorption occurs — causes decreased uptake of calcium, potassium, magnesium, and vitamin D from foods. In time, lack of calcium absorption, particularly during the growing years, can lead to fragile bones that can easily fracture later in life, a condition called osteoporosis. Bones deteriorate

Did You Know?
Gluten-free diet rescue

If celiac disease is diagnosed early and the gluten-free diet is implemented right away, further bone loss and risk of fractures can be prevented. In fact, children following a nutritious, gluten-free diet can usually normalize bone mass within 1 to 2 years.

Once the bone loss has occurred in adults, the research is less clear whether full bone recovery is possible. However, most studies report that major improvements in bone mass are possible if a strict gluten-free diet is followed. Frequently, drug therapy may also be used in addition to dietary measures.

Stages in the progression of osteoporosis

Stage 1: Osteopenia
The first stage in the progression toward osteoporosis is bone loss that reveals low bone mineral density (BMD). There are usually no symptoms associated with osteopenia. Bone mineral density is measured in the hips and spine through an energy X-ray test and is reported as a number called the T-score. Individuals with osteopenia have T-scores of −1.0 to −2.5 standard deviations below the normal.

Stage 2: Onset
Osteoporosis can affect both men and women at any age with undiagnosed celiac disease. In women, menopause accelerates the bone breakdown process by dramatically slowing estrogen production. Osteoporosis is compounded by estrogen loss. Children with undiagnosed celiac disease may develop short stature because they are unable to gain the optimum amount of bone during the period of adolescent bone growth.

Tips for maintaining healthy bones

- Stick to the gluten-free diet — always.
- Get your recommended intake of calcium from dairy and non-dairy foods first; if this doesn't work, your doctor will prescribe calcium and vitamin D supplements along with bone-building drugs.
- Keep active. Weight-bearing exercise, such as jogging, hiking, stair climbing, and resistance training, helps maintain bone mass.
- Eat your veggies. Studies show that fruits and vegetables may protect bone by making the urine more alkaline, but diets high in grains and protein foods generate more acid residues, forcing the body to neutralize it by using calcium from the bones. Fruits and vegetables are also a great source of potassium and vitamin K, which help protect the bone matrix.
- Cut back on salt. A high salt intake causes further calcium loss from bones.
- Moderate your caffeine intake. Caffeine also leads to calcium being lost in the urine.
- Alcohol intake and smoking are additional risk factors for osteoporosis.
- Take vitamin D to assist calcium absorption and to prevent rickets and osteomalacia (softening of the bones).

further in response to cytokines, substances released into the bloodstream by the inflamed intestine. Studies indicate that the autoimmune processes that damage the intestine in celiac disease also attack the bones.

Vitamin D deficiency

Bioactive vitamin D is a steroid hormone that has long been known for its important role in regulating body levels of calcium and phosphorus and in mineralization of bone. Vitamin D is also linked to prevention of colon, prostate, and breast cancers. Evidence from in vitro, animal, and epidemiologic studies shows that vitamin D could play an important role in prevention of type 1 and type 2 diabetes, hypertension, glucose intolerance, and multiple sclerosis. Unfortunately, people with celiac disease are often deficient in vitamin D because of lack of exposure to the sun, low levels in their diet, and malabsorption in the gut.

Recommended vitamin D intake by age group	
Age Group	Adequate Intakes (mcg or IU/day)
Birth–13 years	5 mcg/200 IU
14–18 years (women)	5 mcg/200 IU
14–18 years (men)	5 mcg/200 IU
19–50 years (women)	5 mcg/200 IU
19–50 years (men)	5 mcg/200 IU
51–70 years (women)	10 mcg/400 IU
51–70 years (men)	10 mcg/400 IU
71+ years (women and men)	15 mcg/600 IU
Pregnancy, 14–50 years	5 mcg/200 IU
Lactation, 14–50 years	5 mcg/200 IU

(Source: Institute of Medicine, Food and Nutrition Board, Dietary Reference Intakes: Calcium, Phosphorus, Magnesium, Vitamin D, and Fluoride, 1997.)

Adequate intake of vitamin D

There is a growing body of research regarding the benefits of vitamin D for improving bone health and for preventing cancer, heart disease, and inflammatory bowel disease. This has prompted Health Canada and the Institute of Medicine of the National Academies to review the emerging scientific literature to evaluate whether the current Dietary Reference Intakes (DRIs) need to be revised. For vitamin D, the expert committee will focus on (1) effects of circulating concentrations of 25(OH)D on health outcomes; (2) effects of vitamin D intakes on circulating 25(OH)D and on health outcomes; and (3) levels of intake associated with adverse effects. A report updating the appropriate DRIs for vitamin D and calcium will be issued soon.

Sources of vitamin D

The skin contains a vitamin D precursor that is activated by ultraviolet light to become previtamin D_3, which then needs the assistance of the liver and the kidneys to fully convert to bioactive vitamin D_3. Vitamin D is also available in specific foods and supplements. Like all other fat-soluble vitamins, it is absorbed in the small intestine. Because it is fat-soluble, vitamin D requires some fat for absorption.

Causes of vitamin D deficiency

- **Limited sun exposure.** There are many factors that hinder ultraviolet light from reaching the skin, including cloud cover, shade, sunglasses, and sunscreen. Long winter seasons, living in northern latitudes, and lack of outdoor play are also factors that contribute to the gap in vitamin D stores.

- **Poor diet.** Prolonged exclusive breastfeeding without vitamin D supplementation is a significant cause of rickets, especially in infants whose mothers are already vitamin D deficient.

- **Impaired fat absorption.** Fat malabsorption may be the result of liver or gallbladder disease, cystic fibrosis, gastric bypass, Crohn's disease, or celiac disease.

Rickets

Rickets is a form of vitamin D deficiency most often seen in children whose bones fail to mineralize, resulting in soft bones and deformities. Drinking vitamin D–fortified dairy or non-dairy beverages along with eating vitamin D–fortified foods can completely reverse the effects of rickets.

Osteomalacia

This is the adult form of rickets. Symptoms are subtle, taking a long time to identify, and are characterized by bone pain and muscle weakness.

Food sources of vitamin D

The American and Canadian populations are largely dependent on fortified foods and dietary supplements to meet their vitamin D needs during times of insufficient sunlight, because foods that are naturally rich in vitamin D are not frequently consumed. Natural concentrations of vitamin D in foods vary. Fatty fish represent the richest natural source of vitamin D, with salmon being the type most commonly consumed in North America. Liver and other organ meats are also high in vitamin D but are not as popular as fish and are often avoided because of their high cholesterol content. Although mushrooms and egg yolks are listed as sources of vitamin D, the concentrations are often very low and variable, which results in poor documentation of the vitamin D content of these foods. Fortified fluid milk and breakfast cereals are the predominant vehicles for vitamin D in the United States, whereas Canada fortifies fluid milk and margarine.

Vitamin D content of common foods

The following bar graph outlines food sources of vitamin D, ranked from richest to poorest.

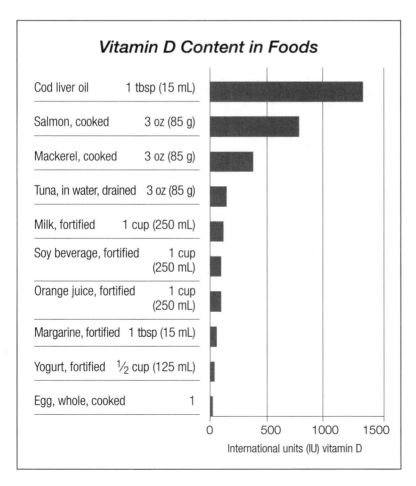

Vitamin D Content in Foods

Supplemental sources of vitamin D

In supplements and fortified foods, vitamin D is available in two forms, D_2 (ergocalciferol) and D_3 (cholecalciferol). The two forms have traditionally been regarded as equivalent, based on their ability to cure rickets, but evidence has been offered that vitamin D_3 could be more than three times as effective as vitamin D_2 in raising blood concentration of vitamin D and maintaining those levels for longer. All vitamin D supplements are gluten-free.

Anemia

Iron is an extremely important mineral for its role in transporting oxygen from the lungs to all body tissues. Oxygen is essential to the way cells generate energy, much as an automobile engine needs oxygen to operate. While iron is not rare in nature, many people, particularly women, do not eat enough iron-containing foods to support their health optimally. In fact, iron deficiency is a problem for millions of people, young and old, male and female, whether they have celiac disease or not.

Symptoms of anemia

The term "anemia" refers to a severe depletion of iron stores, which results in low hemoglobin (red blood cell) concentration. The red blood cells in people with anemia are lighter red and smaller than normal. They cannot carry enough oxygen from

---

Factors affecting iron absorption

- **Forms of iron:** Iron is found in two forms, heme and non-heme. The term "heme" is derived from "hemoglobin," meaning red blood cells. Any food containing muscle and red blood cells will deliver heme iron, which happens to be the most bioavailable. Examples of such foods are red meat, pork, poultry, fish, and shellfish. Non-heme iron is found in legumes, dark leafy greens, and dried fruits.

- **Absorption rate:** Heme iron is more efficiently absorbed than non-heme iron. Healthy people with adequate iron stores absorb heme iron at a relatively constant rate of 23%. However, the rate of absorption for non-heme iron ranges from 2% to 20%, depending on dietary factors and iron stores. People with severe iron deficiency absorb both heme and non-heme iron more efficiently and are more sensitive to dietary enhancing factors than those with better iron status.

---

the lungs to the tissues, so energy release in the cells is hindered. The effect is felt by all the tissues in the body, which explains the feelings of overall fatigue, weakness, headaches, apathy, and poor tolerance to cold. Many of these symptoms may be easily mistaken for behavioral or motivational problems. Stories abound of children who were restless and cranky prior to being diagnosed with celiac disease, or of women who would have to push themselves through the day to complete seemingly simple tasks, only to blame themselves for being lazy.

Iron absorption in celiac disease

In a person with undiagnosed celiac disease, the autoimmune response triggered by the presence of gluten in the intestine destroys the villi lining the proximal duodenum. This is the site of iron absorption.

Recommended iron intake by age group	
Age Group	**Recommended Dietary Allowance (mg/day)**
0–6 months	0.27*
7–12 months	11
1–3 years	7
4–8 years	10
9–13 years (girls)	8
9–13 years (boys)	8
14–18 (women)	15
14–18 years (men)	11
19–30 years (women)	18
19–30 years (men)	8
31–50 years (women)	18
31–50 years (men)	8
51–70 years (men and women)	8
70+ years	8
Pregnancy, 14–50 years	27
Lactation, 14–18 years	10
Lactation, 19–50 years	9

* Denotes adequate intake, which is the mean intake for this age group.

(Source: Institute of Medicine, Food and Nutrition Board, Dietary Reference Intakes: Calcium, Phosphorus, Magnesium, Vitamin D, and Fluoride, 2001.)

Iron content of common foods

The bar graph on page 109 ranks the iron content of common foods from richest to poorest.

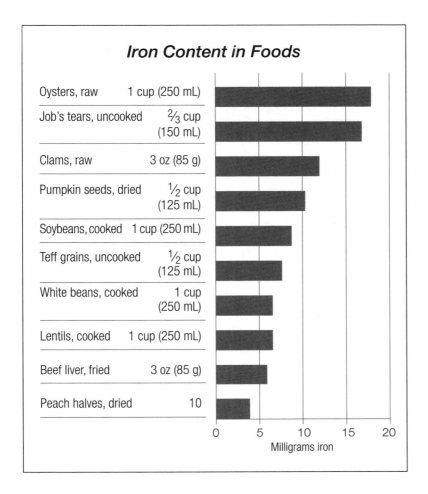

Iron Content in Foods

Food	Amount
Oysters, raw	1 cup (250 mL)
Job's tears, uncooked	2/3 cup (150 mL)
Clams, raw	3 oz (85 g)
Pumpkin seeds, dried	1/2 cup (125 mL)
Soybeans, cooked	1 cup (250 mL)
Teff grains, uncooked	1/2 cup (125 mL)
White beans, cooked	1 cup (250 mL)
Lentils, cooked	1 cup (250 mL)
Beef liver, fried	3 oz (85 g)
Peach halves, dried	10

Milligrams iron (0, 5, 10, 15, 20)

Folate and vitamin B_{12} deficiencies

Folate and vitamin B_{12} are part of a larger group of water-soluble B vitamins that includes thiamin, riboflavin, niacin, biotin, and pantothenic acid. Their roles intertwine because each depends on the other for activation. Together, folate and vitamin B_{12} help cells to multiply, which is very important to cells that must replace themselves quickly. These cells include red blood cells and the cells lining the GI tract — both of which help to deliver energy to all the others. This is why both vitamins — but in particular folate — are so important during the early stages of conception and pregnancy. At this time there is an increased need for new and more red blood cells to carry needed nutrients for proper development. In addition, vitamin B_{12} is responsible for maintaining the sheath that surrounds and protects nerve fibers and promotes their normal growth. Bone cell activity and metabolism also seem to depend on vitamin B_{12}.

Did You Know?
Folate or folic acid supplements

"Folate" is the term used to describe this B vitamin in foods. When taken as a supplement, it is called folic acid. This vitamin is better absorbed from supplements than it is from foods.

Dietary requirements

The dietary requirement for folic acid from supplements during pregnancy has been set at 400 micrograms. The Institute of Medicine has established a tolerable upper intake level (UL) for folate from fortified foods or supplements (folic acid) for ages 1 and above. Intakes above this level increase the risk of adverse health effects. In adults, supplemental folic acid should not

Recommended folate intake by age group

Age Group	Recommended Dietary Allowance (mg/day)
0–6 months	65*
7–12 months	80*
1–3 years	150
4–8 years	200
9–13 years (girls)	300
9–13 years (boys)	300
14–70 years (women)	400
14–70 years (men)	400
71+ years (women)	400
71+ years (men)	400
Pregnancy, 14–50 years	600
Lactation, 14–50 years	500

* There is insufficient information on folate to establish an RDA for infants. An adequate intake (AI) has been established that is based on the amount of folate consumed by healthy infants who are fed breast milk.

(Source: Institute of Medicine, Food and Nutrition Board, Dietary Reference Intakes: Calcium, Phosphorus, Magnesium, Vitamin D, and Fluoride, 1997.)

exceed the UL, to prevent folic acid from triggering symptoms of vitamin B_{12} deficiency. It is important to recognize that the UL refers to the amount of synthetic folate (folic acid) being consumed per day from fortified foods and/or supplements. There is no health risk, and no UL, for natural sources of folate found in food. For adults aged 19 years and older, the UL for folic acid is 1,000 micrograms, or 1 milligram.

Recommended vitamin B_{12} intake by age group

Age Group	Recommended Dietary Allowance (mg/day)
0–6 months	0.4*
7–12 months	0.5*
1–3 years	0.9
4–8 years	1.2
9–13 years (girls)	1.8
9–13 years (boys)	1.8
14–70 years (women)	2.4
14–70 years (men)	2.4
71+ years (women)	2.4
71+ years (men)	2.4
Pregnancy, 14–50 years	2.6
Lactation, 14–50 years	2.8

* There is insufficient information on vitamin B_{12} to establish an RDA for infants. An adequate intake (AI) has been established that is based on the amount of vitamin B_{12} consumed by healthy infants who are fed breast milk.

(Source: Institute of Medicine, Food and Nutrition Board, Dietary Reference Intakes: Calcium, Phosphorus, Magnesium, Vitamin D, and Fluoride, 1997.)

Folate and vitamin B_{12} deficiencies in celiac disease

In celiac disease, damage to the intestinal lining causes malabsorption of both vitamins. Folate is absorbed in the early (proximal) part of the small intestine, while vitamin B_{12} is absorbed from the terminal part of the small intestine (ileum). In addition, vitamin B_{12} requires a protein, called intrinsic factor, in order to be absorbed. When folate, iron, and vitamin B_{12} are poorly absorbed, anemia develops. It is extremely important that your family physician assess you for all three types.

Although a growing number of gluten-free foods are being fortified, there are no mandated requirements for universal fortification of flours and cereal grain products similar to those for mainstream food items. To improve your folic acid and vitamin B_{12} intake, you will need to select foods rich in these vitamins and take supplements.

Types of anemia

- **Megaloblastic anemia:** Because folate and vitamin B_{12} are required to make red blood cells, a deficiency in either one of these nutrients is best diagnosed by looking at hemoglobin levels.

- **Pernicious anemia:** Pernicious anemia is caused by a lack of intrinsic factor, the protein needed to absorb vitamin B_{12}.

- **Iron deficiency anemia:** This kind of anemia is caused by a severe iron deficiency, which affects hemoglobin levels.

Folate and vitamin B_{12} content of common foods

The bar graphs on page 113 show the folate and vitamin B_{12} content in foods commonly eaten, ranked from richest to poorest.

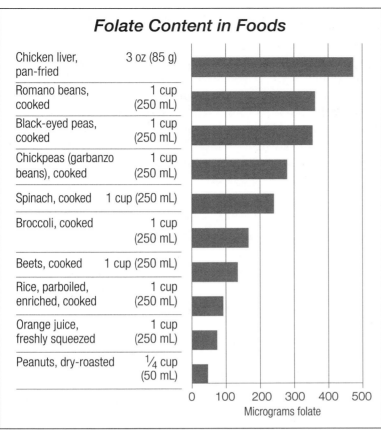

Folate Content in Foods

Food	Amount
Chicken liver, pan-fried	3 oz (85 g)
Romano beans, cooked	1 cup (250 mL)
Black-eyed peas, cooked	1 cup (250 mL)
Chickpeas (garbanzo beans), cooked	1 cup (250 mL)
Spinach, cooked	1 cup (250 mL)
Broccoli, cooked	1 cup (250 mL)
Beets, cooked	1 cup (250 mL)
Rice, parboiled, enriched, cooked	1 cup (250 mL)
Orange juice, freshly squeezed	1 cup (250 mL)
Peanuts, dry-roasted	1/4 cup (50 mL)

Micrograms folate

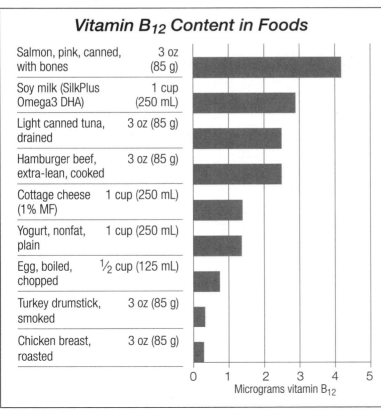

Vitamin B$_{12}$ Content in Foods

Food	Amount
Salmon, pink, canned, with bones	3 oz (85 g)
Soy milk (SilkPlus Omega3 DHA)	1 cup (250 mL)
Light canned tuna, drained	3 oz (85 g)
Hamburger beef, extra-lean, cooked	3 oz (85 g)
Cottage cheese (1% MF)	1 cup (250 mL)
Yogurt, nonfat, plain	1 cup (250 mL)
Egg, boiled, chopped	1/2 cup (125 mL)
Turkey drumstick, smoked	3 oz (85 g)
Chicken breast, roasted	3 oz (85 g)

Micrograms vitamin B$_{12}$

Fiber deficiency

If you fail to eat enough fiber, you will experience gastrointestinal discomfort and constipation. You will also be at a higher risk for developing diverticulosis, colon cancer, heart disease, and a host of other associated diseases. But also beware of eating too much fiber, which can limit or bind the absorption of some nutrients. The amount of fiber you need varies depending on your age, gender, and overall caloric intake. If you adopt a healthy gluten-free diet, you should have no more difficulty meeting your fiber requirements than anyone on a regular diet.

Recommended fiber intake by age group	
Age Group	**Adequate Intake (g/day)**
0–12 months	Not determined
1–3 years	19
4–8 years	25
9–13 years (girls)	26
9–13 years (boys)	31
14–18 years (women)	26
14–18 years (men)	38
19–50 years (women)	25
19–50 years (men)	38
50+ (women)	21
50+ (men)	30
Pregnancy, 14–50 years	28
Lactation, 14–50 years	29

(*Source:* Institute of Medicine, Food and Nutrition Board, *Dietary Reference Intakes: Fibers*, 1997.)

Fiber and celiac disease

Consuming enough fiber is very important for people with celiac disease. Once the gluten-free diet is initiated, many people instinctively reach out for the most obvious gluten-free grains: rice and corn. Potatoes are added to the mix. So are gluten-free baking mixes, most of which use refined flours that have very little remaining fiber and nutrients, unless the product is fortified. In time, if you rely on these foods and shy away from fruits, vegetables, and legumes, the lack of fiber may result in bloating and constipation. To alleviate these symptoms, you need to start by gradually reintroducing small amounts of fiber from gluten-free whole grains, fruits, vegetables, legumes, nuts, and seeds.

Gluten-free foods high in fiber

This graph shows fiber in gluten-free foods, ranked from richest to poorest.

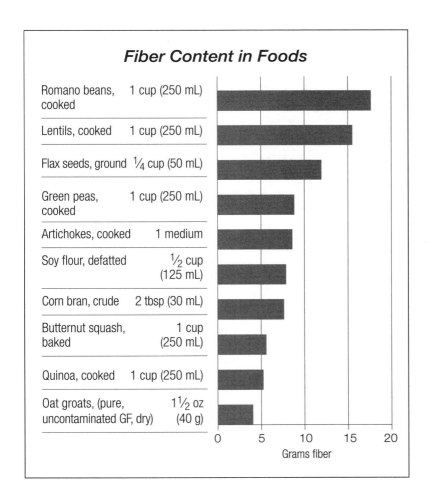

Tips for introducing fiber into your diet

When trying to increase the amount of fiber in your diet, most health professionals recommend introducing it slowly and gradually. Why? Fibers are to the digestive tract what weights are to the muscles. After all, you would not go to the gym and start lifting 30-pound (14 kg) weights on your first visit!

- Start with 15 grams and follow this schedule for 1 month:
  Week 1: 15–20 g (Day 1: 15 g – Day 7: 20 g)
  Week 2: 20–25 g
  Week 3: 25–30 g
  Week 4: 30–35 g
- Choose from among these fiber sources:

	Week 1	Week 2	Week 3	Week 4
Grains servings	4	5	6	7
Fruit servings	1	2	2	3
Vegetables servings	3	3	4	5
Cooked legumes servings	—	½ cup (125 mL)	½ to ¾ cup (125 to 175 mL)	¾ cup (175 mL)

- When increasing fiber, remember to increase your daily fluid intake — up to 6 to 8 cups (1.5 to 2 L) per day. Water is the best choice, but tea, coffee, milk, clear-broth soups, juice, and fruits such as oranges and cantaloupe also count.

Food Guides

While most of us realize that eating habits affect our health, we obviously do not choose foods for their nutritional value only. There are many reasons for making our food choices, such as habits, personal preference, ethnic heritage or tradition, emotional comfort, and availability, convenience, and economics. The trick is to combine favorite foods with fun times as part of a nutritionally balanced gluten-free diet. To help you achieve this balance, consult the *MyPyramid* food guide issued by the United States Department of Agriculture (USDA) and *Eating Well with Canada's Food Guide*, issued by Health Canada. Health Canada also issues a food guide for vegetarians.

These daily food guides are a perfect tool for people with celiac disease to help build a diet that offers

- adequate intake of all nutrients
- balance of essential vitamins and minerals
- calorie control
- nutritionally dense foods
- moderation
- variety

Just remember to choose gluten-free options and substitutes.

USDA MyPyramid Food Guide

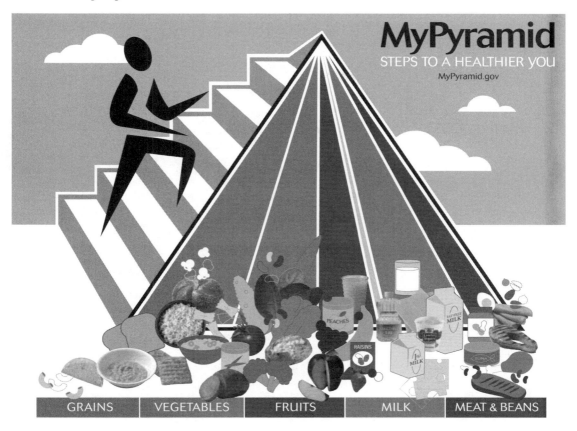

MyPyramid
STEPS TO A HEALTHIER YOU
MyPyramid.gov

GRAINS	VEGETABLES	FRUITS	MILK	MEAT & BEANS

GRAINS Make half your grains whole	VEGETABLES Vary your veggies	FRUITS Focus on fruits	MILK Get your calcium-rich foods	MEAT & BEANS Go lean with protein
Eat at least 3 oz. of whole-grain cereals, breads, crackers, rice, or pasta every day 1 oz. is about 1 slice of bread, about 1 cup of breakfast cereal, or ½ cup of cooked rice, cereal, or pasta	Eat more dark-green veggies like broccoli, spinach, and other dark leafy greens Eat more orange vegetables like carrots and sweetpotatoes Eat more dry beans and peas like pinto beans, kidney beans, and lentils	Eat a variety of fruit Choose fresh, frozen, canned, or dried fruit Go easy on fruit juices	Go low-fat or fat-free when you choose milk, yogurt, and other milk products If you don't or can't consume milk, choose lactose-free products or other calcium sources such as fortified foods and beverages	Choose low-fat or lean meats and poultry Bake it, broil it, or grill it Vary your protein routine — choose more fish, beans, peas, nuts, and seeds

For a 2,000-calorie diet, you need the amounts below from each food group. To find the amounts that are right for you, go to MyPyramid.gov.

Eat 6 oz. every day	Eat 2½ cups every day	Eat 2 cups every day	Get 3 cups every day; for kids aged 2 to 8, it's 2	Eat 5½ oz. every day

Find your balance between food and physical activity
- Be sure to stay within your daily calorie needs.
- Be physically active for at least 30 minutes most days of the week.
- About 60 minutes a day of physical activity may be needed to prevent weight gain.
- For sustaining weight loss, at least 60 to 90 minutes a day of physical activity may be required.
- Children and teenagers should be physically active for 60 minutes every day, or most days.

Know the limits on fats, sugars, and salt (sodium)
- Make most of your fat sources from fish, nuts, and vegetable oils.
- Limit solid fats like butter, stick margarine, shortening, and lard, as well as foods that contain these.
- Check the Nutrition Facts label to keep saturated fats, trans fats, and sodium low.
- Choose food and beverages low in added sugars. Added sugars contribute calories with few, if any, nutrients.

MyPyramid.gov
STEPS TO A HEALTHIER YOU

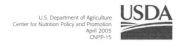

U.S. Department of Agriculture
Center for Nutrition Policy and Promotion
April 2005
CNPP-15

Eating Well with Canada's Food Guide

Recommended Number of *Food Guide Servings* per Day

	Children			Teens		Adults			
Age in Years	2-3	4-8	9-13	14-18		19-50		51+	
Sex	Girls and Boys			Females	Males	Females	Males	Females	Males
Vegetables and Fruit	4	5	6	7	8	7-8	8-10	7	7
Grain Products	3	4	6	6	7	6-7	8	6	7
Milk and Alternatives	2	2	3-4	3-4	3-4	2	2	3	3
Meat and Alternatives	1	1	1-2	2	3	2	3	2	3

What is One Food Guide Serving?
Look at the examples below.

Fresh, frozen or canned vegetables
125 mL (½ cup)

Bread
1 slice (35 g)

Bagel
½ bagel (45 g)

Milk or powdered milk (reconstituted)
250 mL (1 cup)

Cooked fish, shellfish, poultry, lean meat
75 g (2 ½ oz.)/125 mL (½ cup)

The chart above shows how many Food Guide Servings you need from each of the four food groups every day.

Having the amount and type of food recommended and following the tips in *Canada's Food Guide* will help:

• Meet your needs for vitamins, minerals and other nutrients.
• Reduce your risk of obesity, type 2 diabetes, heart disease, certain types of cancer and osteoporosis.
• Contribute to your overall health and vitality.

For a full guide, please contact Health Canada or visit their website.

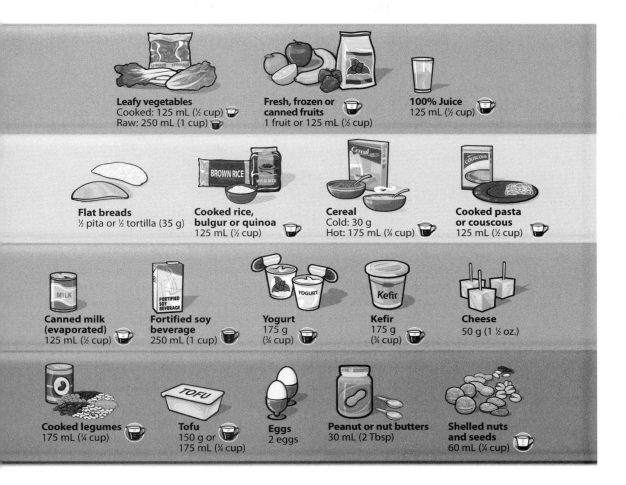

Leafy vegetables
Cooked: 125 mL (½ cup)
Raw: 250 mL (1 cup)

Fresh, frozen or canned fruits
1 fruit or 125 mL (½ cup)

100% Juice
125 mL (½ cup)

Flat breads
½ pita or ½ tortilla (35 g)

Cooked rice, bulgur or quinoa
125 mL (½ cup)

Cereal
Cold: 30 g
Hot: 175 mL (¾ cup)

Cooked pasta or couscous
125 mL (½ cup)

Canned milk (evaporated)
125 mL (½ cup)

Fortified soy beverage
250 mL (1 cup)

Yogurt
175 g
(¾ cup)

Kefir
175 g
(¾ cup)

Cheese
50 g (1 ½ oz.)

Cooked legumes
175 mL (¾ cup)

Tofu
150 g or
175 mL (¾ cup)

Eggs
2 eggs

Peanut or nut butters
30 mL (2 Tbsp)

Shelled nuts and seeds
60 mL (¼ cup)

Oils and Fats

- Include a small amount – 30 to 45 mL (2 to 3 Tbsp) – of unsaturated fat each day. This includes oil used for cooking, salad dressings, margarine and mayonnaise.
- Use vegetable oils such as canola, olive and soybean.
- Choose soft margarines that are low in saturated and trans fats.
- Limit butter, hard margarine, lard and shortening.

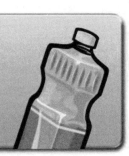

Canada's Food Guide for Vegetarians

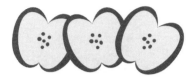

Vegetarian food guide rainbow

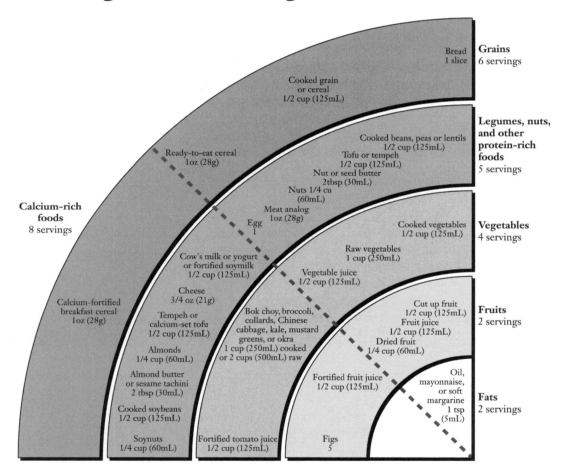

Source: Figure 2 - A new food guide for North American vegetarians. Messina V, Melina V, Mangels AR. *Can Diet Pract Res.* 2003; 64(2):82. (www.dietitians.ca/news/downloads/Vegetarian_Food_Guide_for_NA.pdf) Copyright 2003. Dietitians of Canada. Used with permission.

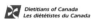
Dietitians of Canada
Les diététistes du Canada

Meal-planning tips

Here are some meal-planning tips for ensuring good nutrition, derived from the chief food guides and adapted for people with celiac disease. Meal-by-meal menus for 4 weeks are presented in the next chapter, followed by gluten-free recipes.

1. **Eat a variety of fruits and vegetables.** The impact of fruits and vegetables on your health, immunity, and overall well-being cannot be overemphasized. Besides the vitamins (B vitamins, vitamin C, vitamin E), minerals (potassium, magnesium) and fiber, fruits and vegetables add beautiful colors and bold textures to your meals. Try to have at least one dark green and one orange vegetable a day.

   Serving = 1 cup (250 mL) raw or $\frac{1}{2}$ cup (125 mL) cooked

2. **Choose whole grains more often.** Make at least half your grain products whole-grain each day. Whole grains provide you with many nutrients, especially B vitamins (thiamin, riboflavin, niacin, and folate), iron, zinc, magnesium, and fiber. These nutrients work together to help provide you with the energy you need to live life fully.

   Serving = $\frac{1}{2}$ cup (125 mL) cooked gluten-free whole grains, 1 slice (35–40 g) gluten-free bread, 1 oz (30 g) gluten-free cold cereal, $\frac{3}{4}$ cup (175 mL) gluten-free whole-grain hot cereal

3. **Drink 2 cups (500 mL) low-fat milk or fortified non-dairy milk each day.** Drinking low-fat milk is a great way to take in protein, calcium, magnesium, riboflavin, vitamin A, vitamin B_{12}, vitamin D, and zinc while minimizing the amount of saturated fat and calories. Fortified soy, rice, and other non-dairy milks are excellent alternatives to regular milk. Make sure that these milks are fortified with vitamin D and, of course, that they are gluten-free.

   Serving = 1 cup (250 mL)

4. **Choose meat alternatives such as beans, lentils, and tofu more often.** Beans, lentils, and tofu provide important nutrients — iron, zinc, magnesium, and B vitamins (thiamin, riboflavin, niacin, vitamin B_6, and vitamin B_{12}). Beans and lentils make you feel satiated because they provide an excellent source of protein and fiber and very little fat — a good choice if you want to lose weight and lower your cholesterol levels.

   Serving = $\frac{3}{4}$ cup (175 mL) cooked legumes or tofu

5. **Eat 2 servings of fish each week.** All fish contain at least some omega-3 essential fatty acids, including EPA (eicosapentaenoic acid) and DHA (docosahexaenoic acid). People should get these fats through food because very little is produced by our bodies. Char, herring, mackerel, rainbow trout, salmon, and sardines have very high amounts of these omega-3 fats. By themselves, EPA and DHA do not account for all the health benefits associated with regularly eating fish. It is likely that the omega-3 fats, the other nutrients found in fish, and the displacement of high-fat foods also contribute to cardiovascular benefits.

   Serving = $2^1/_2$ oz (75 g) cooked fish, poultry, or lean meat, $^1/_4$ cup (60 mL) nuts or seeds, 2 tbsp (30 mL) nut or seed butters

6. **Introduce small amounts of unsaturated fat each day.** Aim for 2 to 3 tbsp (30 to 45 mL) of unsaturated fat from vegetable oils, salad dressings and soft margarines that are low in saturated and trans fats. Reducing your intake of saturated fat and cholesterol is very important to your overall health. What's more, replacing these fats with the healthy alternatives of olive, grapeseed, canola, and other vegetable oils can significantly reduce your risk of heart disease. Healthy fats are also found in nuts and seeds, avocado, fatty fish, and non-hydrogenated margarines.

   Serving = 1 tsp (5 mL) vegetable oil, 2 tsp (10 mL) vinaigrette or fat-reduced mayonnaise

7. **Limit intake of foods with added sugar and added salt.** Sugar and salt are fine in moderation, but the reality is that most processed packaged foods contain more of these additives than we would like to believe. High salt intake is linked to bone loss, and there is increasing evidence that it may also be associated with hypertension, especially if we are predisposed to it. High sugar intake has been linked to impaired glucose tolerance and heart disease.

Serving sizes

Food and nutrition agencies have established serving sizes for various food items in the three macronutrient categories — protein, carbohydrates, and fats. Use these measurements as a guide when preparing a meal for yourself ("Serves 1"), your family, and guests. You can also check to be sure you are not eating more or less food than recommended to maintain good health.

1 Serving =

Carbohydrate Foods

Grains

- 1 slice bread
- ¼ bagel
- ½ cup (125 mL) cooked rice, quinoa, millet, polenta (cornmeal), teff
- ⅓ cup (75 mL) cooked gluten-free pasta
- about 1 oz (30 g) gluten-free cold cereal
- ¾ cup (175 mL) gluten-free hot cereal
- 2 medium rice cakes
- ½ corn tortilla
- 2 cups (500 mL) popcorn

Fruits and vegetables

- 1 medium fruit (apple, orange, peach)
- ½ cup (125 mL) chopped fruit (chopped pineapple, watermelon)
- ½ cup (125 mL) cooked vegetables
- 1 cup (250 mL) raw vegetables
- ½ potato

Protein Foods

Milk and Milk Alternatives

- 1 cup (250 mL) milk (1% MF or less)
- ¾ cup (175 mL) yogurt (1% MF or less)

Meats and Meat Alternatives

- 2½ oz (75 g) meat, poultry, or fish
- 2 eggs or 2 egg whites
- ¾ cup (175 mL) cooked beans (e.g., chickpeas, lentils)
- 1½ oz (45 g) hard cheese (e.g., low-fat Cheddar)
- ¾ cup (175 mL) firm tofu
- ¼ cup (60 mL) seeds or nuts
- ¾ cup (175 mL) hummus

Fats and Oils

- 1 tsp (5 mL) vegetable oil
- 2 tsp (10 mL) salad dressing
- 2 tbsp (30 mL) nut or seed butter
- 1 tsp (5 mL) margarine or butter

CASE HISTORY
Good management — at last

William is 47 years old with a history of bowel frequency and occasional bouts of constipation going back about 10 years. About 2 years ago he was diagnosed with irritable bowel syndrome and tried to manage his symptoms with diet and alternative medicine.

One year ago, his gastrointestinal symptoms were complicated by the sudden onset of episodes of diarrhea and painful gas. He became lactose intolerant and presented with a slow, steady weight loss of 10 pounds (4.5 kg) during this time. There was a family history of gastrointestinal disorders, of which he had very little knowledge because family members would not openly discuss them. Because of this, he was also uncomfortable talking to his family physician about the changes and just lived with the symptoms for much of the time.

When he finally did go to his family physician, William was advised to manage the irritable bowel syndrome through diet, exercise, and stress management. A few months later he went back reporting a further 5-pound (2.3 kg) weight loss and still unresolved symptoms. At this point, he received a referral to a gastroenterologist, who diagnosed him with celiac disease.

Within a week of his being on the gluten-free diet, William's symptoms improved significantly. He was surprised at how easily he had forgotten what it was like to have "normal bowels" again! He came for an initial counseling session on celiac disease, where we discussed ingredients to avoid or those that needed further investigation by contacting manufacturers. He also needed to implement a menu plan to regain some of the weight while keeping in mind the need for adequate fiber, calcium, and B vitamins. At the 3-month check-up, William reported a 3-pound (1.4 kg) weight gain and resolution of his bowel symptoms.

Part 4

Gluten-Free Meal Plans

About the 30-Day Gluten-Free Meal Plans

The meal plans and recipes that follow are meant to guide you toward achieving balance between the energy you take in from foods — the total daily calories — and the important nutrients that help keep you healthy and energetic.

All of the recipes in this book include healthy ingredients. We took advantage of nutritious flours, such as teff, quinoa, sorghum and brown rice flour, and other grains, nuts and seeds, such as millet grits, ground flax seeds, psyllium husks, walnuts, almonds, cashews and sunflower seeds, to pack a nutritional punch into every tasty bite. We incorporated low-fat dairy products, such as part-skim mozzarella cheese, light ricotta cheese and lactose-free 1% milk, and vegan dairy alternatives, such as soy milk and vegan hard margarine, to help you reduce your overall intake of saturated fats and cholesterol. We also chose low-sodium ingredients and used lots of tasty herbs and natural gluten-free spices to replace the need for salt in seasoning. And of course, we included lots of fruits and vegetables! Above all, the meals are delicious and will be enjoyed by everyone in your family, whether or not they need to follow a gluten-free diet.

Each daily meal plan provides you with foods from all food groups. However, you need not follow the meal plan exactly as it is laid out. Rather, let it be a framework for how to combine meals and how to portion them appropriately to achieve your daily recommended intakes for those components that seem to be missing most in a regular gluten-free diet: fiber, iron, calcium and B vitamins such as folate.

When designing the meal plans, the following criteria were taken into consideration:

1. Calories

The tables below, which are based on the Estimated Energy Requirements (EERs) equations from the Institute of Medicine (IOM) Dietary Reference Intakes macronutrients report (2002), will give you an idea of how much food you should consume on a daily basis. They are calculated by gender, age and activity level for individuals of average height and a BMI of 21.5 for adult females or 22.5 for adult males.

Women Age group	Activity Level		
	Sedentary[1]	Low-Active[2]	Active[3]
Age 19–30	2,000	2,000–2,200	2,400
Age 31–50	1,800	2,000	2,200
Age 51+	1,600	1,800	2,000–2,200

Men Age group	Activity Level		
	Sedentary[1]	Low-Active[2]	Active[3]
Age 19–30	2,400	2,600–2,800	3,000
Age 30–50	2,200	2,400–2,600	2,800–3,000
Age 51+	2,000	2,200–2,400	2,400–2,600

1 **Sedentary:** Describes typical daily living activities such as household tasks, walking to the bus.

2 **Low-active:** Describes typical daily living activities *plus* 30 to 60 minutes of daily moderate activity (e.g., walking at 3 to 4 miles per hour, or 5 to 7 kilometers per hour).

3 **Active:** Describes typical daily living activities *plus* at least 60 minutes of daily moderate activity (e.g., walking at 3 to 4 miles per hour, or 5 to 7 kilometers per hour).

Source: *Dietary Guidelines for Americans 2005*, U.S. Department of Agriculture, Center for Nutrition Policy and Promotion, 2005.

The menus presented on pages 128–136 adhere to a plan that provides, on average, 1,800 to 2,000 calories per day, which is in line with the energy requirements for moderately active women who are 31 and older. If your caloric needs are different, you will need to adjust portion sizes accordingly:

- If you have higher caloric needs, increase the portion sizes for the breakfast, lunch and dinner meals. Where a recipe yields 4 to 6 servings, for example, consume one-quarter of the recipe, rather than one-sixth.
- If you have lower caloric needs, skip one of the snack options. You may also need to cut back on the frequency of evening snacks or after-dinner desserts, depending on your activity level.

In the menus, protein, fat and carbohydrate provide the following percentage of total calories:

- **Protein:** 10% to 35% of total calories (i.e., within the recommended range);
- **Fat:** 20% to 35% of total calories (i.e., within the recommended range for adults);
- **Carbohydrate:** 45% to 65% of total calories. (i.e., within the recommended range)

Source: *Reference Intakes for Energy, Carbohydrates, Fiber, Fat, Protein and Amino Acids (Macronutrients),* National Academy of Sciences, 2002.

2. Fiber

The menu plans were designed to provide at least 90% of the daily recommended intake for fiber — 25 to 35 grams per day — for the majority of individuals. Men typically have higher fiber requirements than women (38 grams per day for men between the ages of 20 and 50).

3. Iron

The menu plans were designed to provide between 75% and 80% of the daily recommended intake for iron for women between 31 and 50. This group has the second-highest requirement for iron (18 mg per day, while pregnant women require 27 mg daily), and women make up the majority of those diagnosed with celiac disease. Men in the same age group need only 8 mg of iron per day. It is important for women to maximize their intake of iron from all food sources.

4. Calcium

The menu plans were designed to provide at least 75% to 95% of the daily recommended intake for calcium (1,000 mg per day) for the majority of individuals. Young men and women, along with men and women over 50, have higher calcium requirements (1,300 mg per day for those between the ages of 9 and 18 and 1,200 mg for those over 50).

5. Vitamin D

The latest research indicates the need for a greater intake of vitamin D than was previously believed necessary. The current recommendations are best achieved through supplementation. While there are many food sources of vitamin D, including cod liver oil, salmon and vitamin D–fortified dairy and soy products, it may not be possible to achieve adequate daily intakes of vitamin D through consumption of these foods alone.

6. Folate

The menu plans were designed to provide at least 60% of the daily recommended intake for folate (400 micrograms per day) for the majority of individuals.

Each daily menu plan provides a slightly different amount of all nutrients. Some days will provide you with more iron and less calcium; some will have a higher proportion of calories from fat, while others will be richer in fiber. What's important is to take account of the average intake of nutrients at the end of each week.

Bon appétit!

30-Day Gluten-Free Meal Plans

50-year-old woman, 5'6", 134 lbs, BMI = 21.6 (based on Dietary Reference Intakes for energy, reference heights/weights)

Activity level: Low-active/moderately active (describes typical daily living activities, plus 30 to 60 minutes of daily moderate activity,such as walking at 3 to 4 mph/5 to 7 km/h)

Recommended caloric intake = **1,800 to 2,000 kcal**

Week 1

	Monday	Tuesday	Wednesday
Breakfast	Top of the Morning Egg Wrap 1 cup (250 mL) coffee or tea with 2 tbsp (30 mL) lactose-free skim milk or non-dairy milk	1 Pineapple Carrot Muffin $\frac{3}{4}$ cup (175 mL) low-fat blueberry yogurt 1 cup (250 mL) coffee or tea with 2 tbsp (30 mL) lactose-free skim milk or non-dairy milk	1 Millet and Flax Muffin Fruity Milkshake 1 cup (250 mL) coffee or tea with 2 tbsp (30 mL) lactose-free skim milk or non-dairy milk
AM Snack	1 serving GF whole-grain cereal (e.g., Enjoy Life) with $\frac{3}{4}$ cup (175 mL) lactose-free skim milk or non-dairy milk	Trail Mix	6 GF multigrain crackers (e.g., Mary's Gone Crackers) 1 oz (28 g) part-skim mozzarella string cheese (1 string)
Lunch	2 Crêpes, each filled with with $1\frac{1}{2}$ oz (45 g) GF deli roast beef, $\frac{1}{2}$ cup (125 mL) chopped spinach and 2 tsp (10 mL) hummus Winter Soup Purée	Pasta with Shrimp and Peas 1 peach	Spinach Salad with Chicken and Mandarin Oranges 2 slices Brown Sandwich Bread
PM Snack	1 oz (30 g) almonds (about 24 nuts 6 dried apricots	1 cup (250 mL) baby carrots White Bean Dip	2 oz (60 g) roasted soy nuts 1 apple
Dinner	Pasta with Shrimp and Peas Everyday Salad 1 Cranberry Cluster 1 cup (250 mL) tea with 2 tbsp (30 mL) lactose-free skim milk or non-dairy milk	Tofu Stir-Fry 1 cup (250 mL) cooked wild and brown rice blend (e.g., Lundberg Farms) 1 Chocolate Chip Cookie 1 cup (250 mL) lactose-free skim milk or non-dairy milk	Lasagna with Meat Sauce Everyday Salad $\frac{1}{2}$ cup (125 mL) frozen vanilla yogurt

Daily Nutritional Analysis

Calories (kcal)	1,667	1,975	1,903
Carbohydrate (g)	208	287	209
Fiber (g)	26	29	34
Protein (g)	73	70	104
Fat (g)	64	65	76
Folate (mcg)	191	185	235
Iron (mg)	14	13	15
Calcium (mg)	866	1,024	1,322

Week 1

	Thursday	Friday	Saturday	Sunday
Breakfast	1 serving fortified GF cold cereal with 1 tbsp (15 mL) unsalted raw pumpkin seeds and ½ cup (125 mL) blueberries and 1 cup (250 mL) lactose-free skim milk or non-dairy milk 1 cup (250 mL) coffee or tea with 2 tbsp (30 mL) lactose-free skim milk or non-dairy milk	1 poached egg 2 slices Brown Sandwich Bread with 2 tsp (10 mL) jam ½ cup (125 mL) calcium-fortified orange juice 1 cup (250 mL) coffee or tea with 2 tbsp (30mL) lactose-free skim milk or non-dairy milk	2 Crêpes with Fruit Filling 1½ cups (375 mL) lactose-free skim milk or non-dairy milk latte	2 fried eggs 3 slices (3 oz/90 g) Canadian bacon 1 Savory Tea Biscuit 1 cup (250 mL) calcium-fortified orange juice
AM Snack	1 slice Cranberry Banana Loaf with ½ cup (125 mL) low-fat plain yogurt	½ oz (15 g) unsalted raw pumpkin seeds and 6 dried apricots		
Lunch	Soup à la Mom 1 square Olive and Herb Flatbread	Zucchini Patties Minestrone	Spinach Quiche with Prosciutto 2 cups (500 mL) chopped romaine lettuce with 2 tbsp (30 mL) GF light Italian salad dressing (e.g. Kraft)	Pasta e Fagioli Everyday Salad
PM Snack	1 fortified GF energy bar	¾ cup (175 mL) edamame	2 sesame rice cakes with 4 tsp (20 mL) apple butter and 1 banana	½ cup (125 mL) cauliflower florets 2 tbsp (30 mL) GF yogurt ranch salad dressing
Dinner	Turkey Fingers Zucchini Patties ½ serving Chickpea Salad 1 Cranberry Cluster 1 cup (250 mL) lactose-free skim milk or non-dairy milk	Pizza-Night Pizza Everyday Salad ½ cup (125 mL) frozen yogurt with ½ cup (125 mL) raspberries	Fatina Sweet Potato Fries Orange and Olive Salad Blueberry and Raspberry Crumble	Spaghetti and Meatballs Peas and Mushrooms 1 Maple Walnut Tart 1 cup (250 mL) tea with 2 tbsp (30 mL) lactose-free skim milk or non-dairy milk

Daily Nutritional Analysis

Calories (kcal)	1,943	1,629	1,887	1,786
Carbohydrate (g)	250	209	231	226
Fiber (g)	33	30	27	29
Protein (g)	105	73	79	77
Fat (g)	64	61	79	65
Folate (mcg)	152	548	285	248
Iron (mg)	17	15	11	16
Calcium (mg)	1,329	832	1,144	1,147

Week 2

	Monday	Tuesday	Wednesday
Breakfast	Chewy Granola with 1/2 cup (125 mL) blueberries and 1 cup (250 mL) low-fat vanilla yogurt 1 cup (250 mL) coffee or tea with 2 tbsp (30 mL) lactose-free skim milk or non-dairy milk	Boiled egg 2 slices Brown Sandwich Bread with 2 tsp (10 mL) jam 1/2 cup (125 mL) calcium-fortified orange juice 1 cup (250 mL) coffee or tea with 2 tbsp (30 mL) lactose-free skim milk or non-dairy milk	1 cup (250 mL) cooked quinoa flakes cereal with 1 tbsp (15 mL) raisins, 1 tbsp (15 mL) flax seeds or Salba seeds, 1 tbsp (15 mL) unsalted raw pumpkin seeds and 1 tsp (5 mL) butter 1/2 cup (125 mL) blueberries 1 cup (250 mL) lactose-free skim milk or non-dairy milk latte
AM Snack	6 walnut halves and 6 dried apricots	Trail Mix 1 apple	2 rounds Baby Bell Light cheese 1/2 cup (125 mL) cucumber slices
Lunch	Tuna Casserole Rapini, Red Pepper and Sun-Dried Tomatoes	1 Baked Salmon Patty Mushroom Casserole	Potato, Leek and Broccoli Soup Meatloaf
PM Snack	1 cup (250 mL) edamame	1 Apricot Oatmeal Muffin 1/2 cup (125 mL) lactose-free skim milk or non-dairy milk	1 square Olive and Herb Flatbread with 1/4 cup (60 mL) hummus
Dinner	Chicken Cacciatore Teff Polenta 1 chopped mango with 1/4 cup (60 mL) extra-light ricotta cheese and 2 tbsp (30 mL) agave syrup	Turkey Sausage and Spiral Pasta Greek Salad Chocolate Pudding	Three-Bean Turkey Chili 2 Popovers 3/4 cup (175 mL) low-fat vanilla yogurt 1/2 cup (125 mL) mango slices

Daily Nutritional Analysis

Calories (kcal)	1,876	1,937	1,828
Carbohydrate (g)	241	249	216
Fiber (g)	34	26	32
Protein (g)	102	76	92
Fat (g)	64	76	66
Folate (mcg)	620	190	332
Iron (mg)	17	14	13
Calcium (mg)	732	1,175	1,092

Week 2

	Thursday	Friday	Saturday	Sunday
Breakfast	1 Strawberry Almond Muffin ½ cup (125 mL) calcium-fortified orange juice 1 cup (250 mL) tea with 2 tbsp (30 mL) lactose-free skim milk or non-dairy milk	Crunchy Granola with ½ cup (125 mL) raspberries and 1 cup (250 mL) low-fat plain yogurt 1 cup (250 mL) herbal tea	Breakfast Burrito 1 cup (250 mL) calcium-fortified orange juice	Eggplant and Avocado Fritatta ½ cup (125 mL) cherry tomatoes 1 slice Brown Sandwich Bread 1 cup (250 mL) calcium-fortified orange juice
AM Snack	½ serving Crunchy Granola 1 cup (250 mL) lactose-free skim milk or non-dairy milk latte	1 Yummy Doodle Muffin 1 apricot		
Lunch	Three-Bean Chili with Turkey 1 serving GF corn tortilla chips (about 18)	Quinoa Salad Niçoise 1 pear	Tuna Patties Stuffed Zucchini 6 GF multigrain crackers (e.g., Mary's Gone Crackers)	1½ servings Chickpea Salad 2 Savory Tea Biscuits
PM Snack	Fruity Milkshake	1 Chocolate Hazelnut Biscotti ½ cup (125 mL) lactose-free chocolate milk or chocolate non-dairy milk	Trail Mix	1 banana with 1 tbsp (15 mL) unsalted natural peanut butter
Dinner	Fish for the Sole Orange and Olive Salad Quinoa Pesto Pilaf 1 Chocolate Chip Brownie	Veal Stew Swiss Chard and Potato Salad ½ cup (125 mL) raspberries and ½ cup (125 mL) blackberries with 2 tbsp (30 mL) pure maple syrup	4 oz (125 g) roast chicken breast Cranberry Mandarin Coleslaw Stuffed Artichokes ½ cup (125 mL) frozen yogurt with 2 tbsp (30 mL) GF semisweet chocolate chips	Grilled Chicken Kabob with ¼ cup (60 mL) GF tzatziki Spinach with Almonds 1 cup (250 mL) cooked long-grain brown rice 1 piece Cake of Goodness with Pear Sauce

Daily Nutritional Analysis

Calories (kcal)	1,794	1,891	1,767	1,987
Carbohydrate (g)	220	272	192	258
Fiber (g)	34	35	26	38
Protein (g)	84	86	102	78
Fat (g)	70	57	68	77
Folate (mcg)	284	210	245	372
Iron (mg)	14	14	12	11
Calcium (mg)	1,382	888	960	1,117

Week 3

	Monday	Tuesday	Wednesday
Breakfast	2 Home-Style Pancakes with 2 tbsp (30 mL) pure maple syrup 1/2 cup (125 mL) raspberries 1 cup (250 mL) lactose-free skim milk or non-dairy milk latte	1 Chunky Blueberry Muffin 1 cup (250 mL) low-fat vanilla yogurt 1 cup (250 mL) coffee or tea with 2 tbsp (30 mL) lactose-free skim milk or non-dairy milk	Top of the Morning Egg Wrap 1/2 cup (125 mL) calcium-fortified orange juice 1 cup (250 mL) coffee or tea with 2 tbsp (30 mL) lactose-free skim milk or non-dairy milk
AM Snack	1 oz (30 g) roasted soy nuts 1 apple	2 tbsp (30 mL) unsalted raw pumpkin seeds and 6 dried apricots	1/2 cup (125 mL) blueberry yogurt 1 slice Cranberry Banana Loaf
Lunch	Chicken, Cranberry and Mango Salad 13 GF multigrain crackers (e.g., Mary's Gone Crackers)	Egg Salad Roll-Up Lentil and Spinach Soup	Baked Salmon Patties Spinach with Almonds 3/4 cup (175 mL) cooked millet
PM Snack	After-School Pizza	2 rounds Baby Bell Light cheese 6 GF seed crackers	1/2 GF fruit and nut bar (e.g., Larabar)
Dinner	Skillet Shepherd's Pie Everyday Salad 1 Chocolate Chip Cookie	Turkey Sausage with Lima Bean Medley 1/2 cup (125 mL) cooked millet with Sage Chips 1/2 cup (125 mL) frozen yogurt	Pasta Carbonara Peas and Mushrooms 1 cup (250 mL) raspberries

Daily Nutritional Analysis

Calories (kcal)	2,005	1,926	2,044
Carbohydrate (g)	264	211	260
Fiber (g)	28	27	29
Protein (g)	96	81	91
Fat (g)	67	85	72
Folate (mcg)	85	375	396
Iron (mg)	12	15	14
Calcium (mg)	932	951	1,322

Week 3

	Thursday	Friday	Saturday	Sunday
Breakfast	1 Apricot Oatmeal Muffin Fruity Milkshake	1 Pineapple Carrot Muffin 1 cup (250 mL) 1% cottage cheese or soy yogurt 1 cup (250 mL) coffee or tea with 2 tbsp (30 mL) lactose-free skim milk or non-dairy milk	Breakfast, Brunch or Dessert Waffle with 2 tbsp (30 mL) pure maple syrup 1/2 cup (125 mL) low-fat vanilla yogurt with 1/2 cup (125 mL) blueberries 1 cup (250 mL) coffee or tea with 2 tbsp (30 mL) lactose-free skim milk or non-dairy milk	2 servings French Toast with 2 tbsp (30 mL) pure maple syrup 2 slices (2 oz/60 g) Canadian bacon 1/2 cup (125 mL) blueberries and 1/2 cup (125 mL) blackberries 1 cup (250 mL) coffee or tea with 2 tbsp (30 mL) lactose-free skim milk or non-dairy milk
AM Snack	1/2 cup (125 mL) GF rice pudding 1 cup (250 mL) grapes	2 tbsp (30 mL) unsalted raw pumpkin seeds and 2 tbsp (30 mL) raisins		
Lunch	4 oz (112 g) canned tuna in water, drained Polenta with Tomato Sauce	Mushroom Casserole Fennel and Sun-Dried Tomatoes	Salsa Burger on a GF hamburger bun with 2 tsp (10 mL) ketchup, 2 tsp (10 mL) prepared mustard (e.g., French's) Sweet Potato Fries Everyday Salad	2 servings Asparagus Wraps Quinoa Salad
PM Snack	1 cup (250 mL) edamame	1 cup (250 mL) baby carrots 2 servings White Bean Dip	1 slice watermelon (1/16 melon)	1 Yummy Doodle Muffin 1/2 cup (125 mL) lactose-free chocolate milk or chocolate non-dairy milk
Dinner	Oven-Baked Beef Stew Potato and Sweet Potato Bake 1 Cranberry Cluster 1 cup (250 mL) tea with 2 tbsp (30 mL) lactose-free skim milk or non-dairy milk	4 oz (125 g) grilled salmon fillet Cranberry Mandarin Coleslaw 1/2 cup (125 mL) cooked wild and brown rice blend (e.g., Lundberg Farms) 2 Almond Cookies 1 cup (250 mL) tea with 2 tbsp (30 mL) lactose-free skim milk or non-dairy milk	Chicken Pot Pie Stuffed Artichokes Chocolate Pudding	Veal Stew over Nokedli 1/2 cup (125 mL) papaya chunks

Daily Nutritional Analysis

Calories (kcal)	1,731	1,956	1,998	1,998
Carbohydrate (g)	206	221	269	233
Fiber (g)	27	35	32	30
Protein (g)	94	99	89	93
Fat (g)	60	78	69	80
Folate (mcg)	566	340	227	230
Iron (mg)	16	18	14	12
Calcium (mg)	1,038	830	976	954

Week 4

	Monday	Tuesday	Wednesday
Breakfast	Chewy Granola with 1 cup (250 mL) lactose-free skim milk or non-dairy milk 1½ cups (375 mL) sliced strawberries 1 cup (250 mL) herbal tea	1 slice Pear and Walnut Loaf 1 serving (6 oz or 200 mL) GF drinkable yogurt (e.g., Yop vanilla) 1 cup (250 mL) coffee or tea with 2 tbsp (30 mL) lactose-free skim milk or non-dairy milk	2 slices Brown Sandwich Bread with 2 tbsp (30 mL) almond butter and 1 tbsp (15 mL) apple butter 1 cup (250 mL) coffee or tea with 2 tbsp (30 mL) lactose-free skim milk or non-dairy milk
AM Snack	½ cup (125 mL) plain or flavored yogurt 5 or 6 pecan and rice crisps (e.g., Nut Thins)	1 oz (28 g) part-skim mozzarella string cheese (1 string) ½ yellow bell pepper, cut into strips	1 Chocolate Hazelnut Biscotti 1 cup (250 mL) lactose-free skim milk or non-dairy milk latte
Lunch	Spinach Salad with Chicken and Mandarin Oranges 1 square Olive and Herb Flatbread	Tuna Patties Lentil and Spinach Soup 1 slice Brown Sandwich Bread	Crustless Rapini and Clam Quiche 2 cups (500 mL) shredded romaine with 2 tbsp (30 mL) GF light raspberry salad dressing 13 GF multigrain crackers (e.g., Mary's Gone Crackers)
PM Snack	20 GF soy crisps (e.g., Glenny's Soy Crisps) 1 apple	1 Zucchini Oatmeal Muffin	1 cup (250 mL) broccoli florets White Bean Dip
Dinner	Spaghetti and Meatballs Everyday Salad 1 Hazelnut Shortbread Cookie 1 cup (250 mL) tea with 2 tbsp (30 mL) lactose-free skim milk or non-dairy milk	Crustless Rapini and Clam Quiche Quinoa Salad ½ cup (125 mL) chopped peaches and ½ cup (125 mL) blackberries, with 1 tbsp (15 mL) pure maple syrup	Turkey Fingers Pizza Topping Stir-Fry 1 cup (250 mL) cooked wild and brown rice blend (e.g., Lundberg Farms) 1 Crêpe with Fruit Filling

Daily Nutritional Analysis

Calories (kcal)	1,884	1,714	1,900
Carbohydrate (g)	267	192	225
Fiber (g)	34	28	32
Protein (g)	85	93	92
Fat (g)	57	69	75
Folate (mcg)	239	398	336
Iron (mg)	14	20	20
Calcium (mg)	978	1,304	1,075

Week 4

	Thursday	Friday	Saturday	Sunday
Breakfast	1 egg, scrambled with 1 slice (1 oz/30 g) Canadian bacon and $\frac{1}{2}$ cup (125 mL) sliced mushrooms 2 slices Brown Sandwich Bread $\frac{1}{2}$ cup (125 mL) calcium-fortified orange juice 1 cup (250 mL) coffee or tea with 2 tbsp (30 mL) lactose-free skim milk or non-dairy milk	French Toast with 2 tbsp (30 mL) pure maple syrup 1 cup (250 mL) blueberries with $\frac{1}{2}$ cup (125 mL) low-fat vanilla yogurt 1 cup (250 mL) herbal tea	Breakfast Burrito $\frac{1}{2}$ cup (125 mL) chopped cantaloupe and $\frac{1}{2}$ cup (125 mL) chopped honeydew melon 1 cup (250 mL) coffee or tea with 2 tbsp (30 mL) lactose-free skim milk or non-dairy milk	2 Home-Style Pancakes with 2 tbsp (30 mL) pure maple syrup 1 cup (250 mL) chopped mango 1 cup (250 mL) lactose-free skim milk or non-dairy milk latte
AM Snack	1 oz (30 g) roasted soy nuts 1 cup (250 mL) grapes	2 wedges Laughing Cow (La Vache Qui Rit) cheese $\frac{1}{4}$ cup (60 mL) cucumber slices 5 cassava crackers		
Lunch	1$\frac{1}{2}$ servings Minestrone 1 Savory Tea Biscuit	Quinoa Salad Niçoise	1 Crêpe with 1 tsp (5 mL) margarine, 2 tsp (10 mL) Dijon mustard, 2 to 3 oz (60 to 90 g) GF deli cooked ham and $\frac{1}{2}$ cup (125 mL) chopped spinach Chickpea Salad	Sardines and Toast Soup à la Mom
PM Snack	1 slice Banana Almond Bread $\frac{1}{2}$ cup (125 mL) low-fat yogurt	Hot Spinach and Broccoli Dip 6 rice and almond crackers (e.g., Nut Thins)	$\frac{1}{2}$ cup (125 mL) 1% cottage cheese 1 cup (250 mL) fresh pineapple chunks	1 apple, cut into slices, with 2 tbsp (30 mL) unsalted natural peanut butter
Dinner	Grilled Chicken Kabob Quinoa Pesto Pilaf Greek Salad $\frac{1}{2}$ cup (125 mL) sorbet	Eggplant and Zucchini Lasagna Everyday Salad Chocolate Pudding	Fish for the Sole Spinach with Almonds 1 cup (250 mL) cooked brown rice couscous (e.g., Lundberg Farms) Blueberry and Raspberry Crumble	Gnocchi with $\frac{1}{2}$ cup (125 mL) GF tomato sauce and 2 tbsp (30 mL) freshly grated Parmesan cheese Green Beans and Romano Cheese 1 cup (250 mL) chopped watermelon

Daily Nutritional Analysis

Calories (kcal)	1,985	1,927	1,718	1,803
Carbohydrate (g)	249	260	219	281
Fiber (g)	25	27	27	31
Protein (g)	98	73	79	62
Fat (g)	71	67	65	53
Folate (mcg)	168	166	347	147
Iron (mg)	14	12	10	11
Calcium (mg)	919	1,184	496	1,306

Week 5

	Monday	Tuesday
Breakfast	1¼ cups (300 mL) GF cereal (e.g., Nature's Path Mesa Sunrise) 1 cup (250 mL) strawberries 1 cup (250 mL) lactose-free skim milk or non-dairy milk 1 cup (250 mL) tea	Spinach Quiche with Prosciutto 1 cup (125 mL) calcium-fortified orange juice 1 cup (250 mL) coffee or tea with 2 tbsp (30 mL) lactose-free skim milk or non-dairy milk
AM Snack	2 tbsp (30 mL) unsalted sunflower seeds 1 orange	1 Pineapple Carrot Muffin
Lunch	Baked Salmon Patties Teff Polenta	2 servings Asparagus Wraps Chickpea Soup 1 slice Brown Sandwich Bread
PM Snack	Crunchy Granola	1 whole-grain brown rice cake (e.g., Lundberg Farms) 2 plums
Dinner	Turkey Sausage and Spiral Pasta Rapini, Red Pepper and Sun-Dried Tomatoes 1 cup (250 mL) cantaloupe balls	Tofu Stir-Fry ¾ cup (175 mL) cooked millet 2 Traditional Tea Biscuits with 2 tsp (10 mL) butter or vegan hard margarine and 2 tsp (10 mL) jam 1 cup (250 mL) tea with 2 tbsp (30 mL) lactose-free skim milk or non-dairy milk

Daily Nutritional Analysis

Calories (kcal)	1,818	1,917
Carbohydrate (g)	252	248
Fiber (g)	36	26
Protein (g)	77	76
Fat (g)	62	76
Folate (mcg)	265	264
Iron (mg)	15	13
Calcium (mg)	933	1,697

Daily Fluid Intake

Water and other fluids are essential for staying hydrated and allowing the body to transport nutrients and get rid of wastes. According to the National Academies of Sciences, total water intake includes drinking water, water in beverages and water that is part of food. Women living in temperate climates need 9 cups (2.2 L) total water daily, while men need 13 cups (3 L) daily. You'll need to consume more if you live in a hot climate or engage in moderate to vigorous activity.

With the exception of alcoholic beverages, all beverages count toward the daily recommended intakes for total water, including coffee, tea, milk, soup, juice and even soft drinks. However, it's best to choose water over juice or soft drinks to satisfy your thirst. The water in fruits, vegetables and other foods also counts, but it is much harder to quantify. Nevertheless, it's a good idea to have fruit and vegetables more often than juice.

Generally, you should aim to drink:

- One to 2 cups (250 to 500 mL) of fluid with each main meal (breakfast, lunch and dinner). If a meal already calls for 1 cup (250 mL) milk, supplement that meal with ½ to 1 cup (125 to 250 mL) water, depending on your thirst.

- At least 1 to 2 cups (250 to 500 mL) of water with mid-morning and mid-afternoon snacks.

Part 5

Healthy Gluten-Free Recipes

Breakfast and Brunch

Crunchy Granola

Alexandra likes to add this granola to yogurt and let it soften for 5 minutes before eating it. She also adds blueberries on top. Yum.

Tips

Make sure the oats you buy are labeled "pure oats" or have a gluten-free certification — this assures you that there has been no cross-contamination with wheat, barley or rye.

Store in an airtight container in a cool, dry place for up to 2 weeks.

- Preheat oven to 300°F (150°C)
- Baking sheet, lined with parchment paper

2 cups	GF large-flake (old-fashioned) rolled oats (see tip, at left)	500 mL
1 cup	kasha (roasted buckwheat groats)	250 mL
½ cup	psyllium husks	125 mL
½ cup	light (fancy) molasses	125 mL
¼ cup	agave nectar	60 mL
½ cup	shredded coconut	125 mL
½ cup	dried cranberries	125 mL
½ cup	dried apricots	125 mL
½ cup	slivered almonds	125 mL
½ cup	unsalted sunflower seeds	125 mL
1 tbsp	ground cinnamon	15 mL

1. In a bowl, combine oats, kasha and psyllium. Stir in molasses and agave nectar. Stir in coconut, cranberries, apricots, almonds, sunflower seeds and cinnamon until well combined.

2. Using a spatula, spread granola evenly on prepared baking sheet. Bake in preheated oven for 15 to 30 minutes or until golden brown and hard. Let cool on baking sheet, then break into pieces.

Psyllium Husks

Psyllium husks are the outer part of psyllium seeds, which are from the plantain plant, *Plantago ovato*. Numerous large-scale studies have shown that daily consumption of small amounts of psyllium fiber (3 to 12 grams a day) can help reduce LDL cholesterol ("bad" cholesterol). Other research indicates that when psyllium is incorporated into food, it is more effective at reducing the blood glucose response than a soluble fiber supplement that is taken separately from food.

Nutrients Per Serving

Calories	300
Carbohydrate	50 g
Fiber	8 g
Protein	6 g
Fat	9 g
Iron	3 mg
Calcium	75 mg

Chewy Granola

Theresa prefers this softer-textured granola. It's great as either a breakfast cereal or a snack.

Tips

Store in an airtight container in the refrigerator for up to 1 week.

For added nutrition, serve with fresh berries.

- Preheat oven to 300°F (150°C)
- Baking sheet, lined with parchment paper

1 cup	GF large-flake (old-fashioned) rolled oats (see tip, page 140)	250 mL
¼ cup	psyllium husks	60 mL
½ cup	unsweetened applesauce	125 mL
¼ cup	pure maple syrup	60 mL
¼ cup	dried cranberries	60 mL
¼ cup	slivered almonds	60 mL
¼ cup	unsalted sunflower seeds	60 mL
¼ cup	sesame seeds	60 mL
1 tsp	ground cinnamon	5 mL

1. In a bowl, combine oats and psyllium. Stir in applesauce and maple syrup. Stir in cranberries, almonds, sunflower seeds, sesame seeds and cinnamon until well combined.

2. Using a spatula, spread granola evenly on prepared baking sheet. Bake in preheated oven for 15 to 30 minutes or until light golden. Let cool on baking sheet, then break into pieces.

Nutrients Per Serving

Calories	210
Carbohydrate	32 g
Fiber	6 g
Protein	5 g
Fat	7 g
Iron	2 mg
Calcium	31 mg

Top of the Morning Egg Wrap

Theresa taught her children how to cook when they were very young, and it was one of her sons who came up with this recipe.

Tips

Look for nitrate-free turkey slices, as they are a healthier alternative.

You can substitute GF Cheddar-style rice cheese or mozzarella-style rice cheese for the Cheddar cheese.

1 tbsp	grapeseed oil	15 mL
4	slices GF deli-roasted turkey (see tip, at left)	4
Dash	GF soy sauce	Dash
4	eggs	4
4	Crêpes (see recipe, page 150)	4
2	romaine lettuce leaves, torn in half	2
1/4 cup	shredded Cheddar cheese	60 mL

1. In a skillet, heat oil over medium-high heat. Add turkey and soy sauce; cook for about 1 minute per side or until golden. Transfer turkey to a plate and set aside.

2. Break eggs into the liquid remaining in skillet, making sure to break the yolks. Cook, turning once, until set on both sides.

3. Place a crêpe on each plate and layer with lettuce, turkey, egg and cheese. Fold or roll up.

Nutrients Per Serving	
Calories	240
Carbohydrate	16 g
Fiber	1 g
Protein	15 g
Fat	13 g
Iron	1 mg
Calcium	67 mg

Breakfast Burrito

These burritos are fantastic for breakfast — or any meal, for that matter. Serve with sliced avocado, tomato and mango.

Tips

You can substitute GF Cheddar-style rice cheese for the Cheddar cheese.

If you already have crêpes made, be sure to microwave them on High for 20 seconds before assembling.

1 tsp	grapeseed oil	5 mL
1½ cups	rinsed drained canned black beans	375 mL
½ cup	salsa	125 mL
¼ cup	chopped drained pickled hot peppers	60 mL
4	eggs, beaten	4
1 cup	shredded Cheddar cheese, divided	250 mL
6	Crêpes (see recipe, page 150)	6

1. In a skillet, heat oil over medium-high heat. Sauté black beans for 3 to 5 minutes or until heated through. Add salsa and hot peppers; sauté for 3 to 5 minutes or until heated through. Add eggs and cook, stirring, until set. Remove from heat and stir in half the cheese.

2. Spoon one-sixth of the egg mixture along the center of each crêpe. Top with the remaining cheese and roll up.

Nutrients Per Serving	
Calories	250
Carbohydrate	28 g
Fiber	5 g
Protein	15 g
Fat	9 g
Iron	2 mg
Calcium	120 mg

Eggplant and Avocado Frittata

Makes 4 servings

Frittata means "fried" in Italian. Theresa loves both eggplant and avocado and decided to put them together in a frittata. The result? Divine.

Tip

Cutting the frittata into four pieces makes it easier to flip.

1½ tbsp	grapeseed oil	22 mL
1 cup	chopped red bell pepper	250 mL
½ cup	chopped onion	125 mL
1 tbsp	chopped fresh parsley	15 mL
2 cups	chopped Japanese eggplant (about 1 medium)	500 mL
4	eggs, beaten	4
½ cup	shredded sharp (old) Cheddar cheese	125 mL
1	avocado, mashed	1
¼ cup	grated Romano cheese	60 mL

1. In a skillet, heat oil over medium heat. Sauté red pepper, onion and parsley for 3 to 5 minutes or until tender. Add eggplant and sauté for 5 to 10 minutes or until soft and golden.

2. Pour eggs over vegetables and cook until edges are firm. Cut into four pieces. Flip each piece over and spread evenly with avocado. Remove from heat and sprinkle cheese evenly over avocado. Cover and let stand for 1 to 2 minutes. Serve hot.

Nutrients Per Serving	
Calories	280
Carbohydrate	12 g
Fiber	6 g
Protein	14 g
Fat	20 g
Iron	1 mg
Calcium	176 mg

Spinach Quiche with Prosciutto

Tip

Choose your favorite GF non-dairy milk, such as soy, rice, almond or potato-based milk or, if you tolerate lactose, use regular 1% milk.

- Preheat oven to 350°F (180°C)
- 9-inch (23 cm) glass pie plate

	Pie Pastry for one 9-inch (23 cm) single-crust pie (see recipe, page 250)	
8 oz	spinach (about 5 cups/1.25 L), trimmed	250 g
4	eggs	4
1 cup	lactose-free 1% milk or fortified GF non-dairy milk	250 mL
2 cups	shredded light Cheddar cheese	500 mL
3 to 4	slices prosciutto, fat removed	3 to 4

1. Fit pie pastry into pie plate. Bake in preheated oven for 10 minutes. Remove from oven, leaving the oven on, and let cool slightly.

2. In a large pot of boiling water, boil spinach for 1 to 2 minutes or until wilted. Drain and set aside.

3. In a bowl, whisk together eggs and milk. Whisk in cheese and drained spinach.

4. Arrange prosciutto on bottom of pie crust. Pour in egg mixture. Bake for 35 to 40 minutes or until puffed and golden brown and a tester inserted in the center comes out clean. Let stand for about 10 minutes before cutting into wedges.

Sardines and Toast

Toast and butter a slice of GF bread, then place a sardine, including the oil it was packed in, on top and spread evenly over the toast. Serve with slices of tomato. Theresa's husband loves this for breakfast.

(Nutrients per serving: Calories: 180; Carbohydrate: 23 g; Fiber: 4 g; Protein: 8 g; Fat: 6 g; Iron: 2 mg; Calcium: 111 mg)

Nutrients Per Serving

Calories	320
Carbohydrate	24 g
Fiber	2 g
Protein	13 g
Fat	16 g
Iron	2 mg
Calcium	347 mg

French Toast

This recipe is so simple and delicious, especially when it's served with blueberries and strawberries on the side.

Tip

Choose your favorite GF non-dairy milk, such as soy, rice, almond or potato-based milk or, if you can tolerate lactose, use regular 1% milk.

Vegan hard margarine, such as Earth Balance vegan buttery flavor sticks, has almost half as much saturated fat as regular butter and no cholesterol. Where butter is called for in a recipe, vegan hard margarine can be a heart-healthy, delicious alternative.

1	egg	1
½ cup	fortified GF non-dairy milk or lactose-free 1% milk	125 mL
½ tsp	vanilla extract	2 mL
4 tsp	butter or vegan hard margarine, divided	20 mL
4	slices stale enriched GF bread, cut in half	4
	Ground cinnamon	
	Pure maple syrup or agave nectar (optional)	

1. In a large flat-bottomed bowl, beat egg, milk and vanilla until frothy.

2. In a skillet, melt 1 tsp (5 mL) of the butter over medium-high heat. Working with two half slices at a time, dip both sides of bread in egg mixture. Transfer to skillet and cook, turning once, for 2 to 3 minutes per side or until browned on both sides. Transfer to a plate and keep warm. Repeat with the remaining bread and egg mixture, melting another 1 tsp (5 mL) butter in the skillet before each batch.

3. Serve sprinkled with cinnamon and drizzled with maple syrup, if desired.

Nutrients Per Serving	
Calories	210
Carbohydrate	23 g
Fiber	4 g
Protein	4 g
Fat	8 g
Iron	1 mg
Calcium	70 mg

Breakfast, Brunch or Dessert Waffles

You might think you have to give up waffles when you learn you have to eat a GF diet, but these waffles are so good you won't believe they're gluten-free. Top them with ice cream and berries as an added treat.

Tips

Depending on your waffle maker, the cooking time could vary from as little as 2 minutes to as much as 5 minutes. Read the manual for your waffle maker and adjust the time accordingly.

Prepare these ahead of time, let them cool, layer with parchment paper and freeze for up to 1 month. Toast them in the morning for a quick breakfast or whenever you crave a waffle.

Nutrients Per Serving

Calories	260
Carbohydrate	28 g
Fiber	2 g
Protein	7 g
Fat	14 g
Iron	1 mg
Calcium	154 mg

- Waffle maker, lightly oiled with grapeseed oil, then preheated

¾ cup	white rice flour	175 mL
¼ cup	sorghum flour	60 mL
¼ cup	potato starch	60 mL
¼ cup	ground flax seeds (flaxseed meal)	60 mL
1 tbsp	GF baking powder	15 mL
¼ tsp	salt	1 mL
2	eggs, separated	2
2 cups	fortified GF non-dairy milk or lactose-free 1% milk (see tip, page 146)	500 mL
¼ cup	grapeseed oil	60 mL

1. In a large bowl, using a whisk, combine white rice flour, sorghum flour, potato starch, flax seeds, baking powder and salt.

2. In another bowl, whisk together egg yolks, milk and oil until blended. Stir into flour mixture until well blended.

3. In a small bowl, using an electric mixer, beat egg whites until stiff. Fold egg whites into batter until just blended. Let stand for 5 minutes.

4. Pour about ¾ cup (175 mL) batter onto prepared hot waffle maker (or the amount appropriate for your waffle maker). Close lid and cook for about 3 minutes (see tip, at left) or until golden brown. Transfer to a plate and keep warm. Repeat with the remaining batter, stirring batter and lightly oiling waffle maker with grapeseed oil between batches as needed.

Home-Style Pancakes

These fantastic pancakes taste just like the ones Mom used to make. Serve topped with fruit and drizzle with maple syrup.

Tip

Choose your favorite GF non-dairy milk, such as soy, rice, almond or potato-based milk or, if you can tolerate lactose, use regular 1% milk.

1/2 cup	sorghum flour	125 mL
1/2 cup	brown rice flour	125 mL
2 tbsp	psyllium husks	30 mL
1 tsp	GF baking powder	5 mL
1/4 tsp	baking soda	1 mL
1/4 tsp	salt	1 mL
1	egg	1
1 cup	fortified GF non-dairy milk or lactose-free 1% milk	250 mL
1 tbsp	liquid honey, pure maple syrup or agave nectar	15 mL
2 tsp	grapeseed oil	10 mL
1 tsp	vanilla extract	5 mL
	Butter or grapeseed oil	

1. In a large bowl, combine sorghum flour, brown rice flour, psyllium, baking powder, baking soda and salt.

2. In another bowl, beat egg, milk, honey, oil and vanilla. Pour into flour mixture and whisk for about 1 minute or until smooth.

3. On a griddle or in a nonstick skillet, melt 1 tsp (5 mL) butter over medium heat. For each pancake, pour in 1/4 cup (60 mL) batter. Cook for 1 to 2 minutes or until bubbles start to form and edges are firm. Flip over and cook other side for 1 to 2 minutes or until bottom is golden. Transfer to a plate and keep warm. Repeat with the remaining batter, greasing griddle and adjusting heat between batches as needed.

Nutrients Per Serving	
Calories	150
Carbohydrate	21 g
Fiber	2 g
Protein	4 g
Fat	5 g
Iron	1 mg
Calcium	127 mg

Variation

Applesauce Pancakes:
Add $\frac{1}{2}$ cup (125 mL) unsweetened applesauce to the batter. The pancakes may take a minute or two longer to cook. Serve sprinkled with chopped walnuts and ground cinnamon, then drizzled with maple syrup.

Time-Saving Tips

Combine the dry ingredients and store in an airtight container for up to 2 weeks.

Cook the pancakes the night before and store them in the refrigerator. Toast them in the morning.

Cooled cooked pancakes can also be placed in an airtight container, with parchment paper between each one for easier separation, and stored in the freezer for up to 4 weeks. Toast to serve.

Psyllium Husks

Psyllium husks are the outer part of psyllium seeds, which are from the plantain plant, *Plantago ovato*. Numerous large-scale studies have shown that daily consumption of small amounts of psyllium fiber (3 to 12 grams a day) can help reduce LDL cholesterol ("bad" cholesterol). Other research indicates that when psyllium is incorporated into food, it is more effective at reducing the blood glucose response than a soluble fiber supplement that is taken separately from food.

Crêpes

These crêpes are so good, it's worth getting up a half-hour early to prepare them. They can be used to make enchiladas or as wraps filled with cream cheese and hot pepper slices, cream cheese and cucumber slices, cashew butter and banana slices, peanut butter and jam — the possibilities are endless.

Tips

Choose your favorite GF non-dairy milk, such as soy, rice, almond or potato-based milk or, if you tolerate lactose, use regular 1% lactose-free milk.

Crêpes can be prepared ahead of time, cooled, layered between sheets of parchment paper and stored in an airtight container in the refrigerator for up to 3 days. Just before serving, reheat each crêpe on a plate in the microwave on High for about 20 seconds to soften it.

Nutrients Per Serving	
Calories	100
Carbohydrate	14 g
Fiber	1 g
Protein	3 g
Fat	4 g
Iron	0.4 mg
Calcium	20 mg

- 9-inch (23 cm) skillet

1/2 cup	sorghum flour	125 mL
1/2 cup	potato starch	125 mL
1/2 tsp	granulated raw cane sugar	2 mL
2	eggs	2
1/2 cup	lactose-free 1% milk or fortified GF non-dairy milk	125 mL
2 tbsp	butter or vegan hard margarine, melted	30 mL
	Butter or vegan hard margarine	

1. In a large bowl, using a whisk, combine sorghum flour, potato starch and sugar.

2. In another bowl, beat eggs, milk, melted butter and 1/2 cup (125 mL) water. Stir into flour mixture until well blended.

3. In skillet, melt 1/2 tsp (2 mL) butter over medium heat, making sure to cover the bottom of the skillet. For each crêpe, pour in a scant 1/4 cup (60 mL) batter and swirl so that the batter covers the whole surface. Cook for about 1 minute or until edges start to curl up. Flip over and cook for 1 minute or until bottom is golden. Transfer to a plate and keep warm. Repeat with the remaining batter, adjusting heat and melting another 1/2 tsp (2 mL) butter between each batch as needed.

Crêpes with Fruit Filling

These yummy fruit-filled crêpes are great for either breakfast or dessert.

Tip

If peaches, strawberries and blueberries are not in season, you can substitute frozen fruit. Thaw it in the skillet over low heat, then continue with step 1, omitting the water.

2 cups	sliced peaches	500 mL
2 cups	sliced strawberries	500 mL
1 cup	blueberries	250 mL
2 tsp	agave nectar	10 mL
1 tsp	white rice flour	5 mL
4	Crêpes (see recipe, page 150)	4

1. In a skillet, combine peaches, strawberries, blueberries and 2 tbsp (30 mL) water. Drizzle with agave nectar and rice flour; cook over low heat, stirring gently, for 3 to 5 minutes or until thickened.

2. Spoon filling down the center of each crêpe and roll up or fold.

Nutrients Per Serving	
Calories	190
Carbohydrate	36 g
Fiber	4 g
Protein	4 g
Fat	5 g
Iron	1 mg
Calcium	40 mg

Fruity Milkshake

Makes 3 servings

Pour this delicious shake into a stainless steel container and enjoy it on your way to work or as a pick-me-up snack. In the summer, Theresa pours it into ice pop containers and freezes it for a refreshing treat the kids love! By all means, double or triple this recipe to make as much as you need.

Tip

You can purchase ground flax seeds (which may be called flaxseed meal), grind whole seeds in the blender before adding the remainder of the ingredients, or grind them in a coffee or spice grinder. If you grind your own, ensure that your blender, coffee grinder or spice grinder is used for gluten-free foods only, to avoid the risk of cross-contamination.

Nutrients Per Serving	
Calories	120
Carbohydrate	18 g
Fiber	3 g
Protein	5 g
Fat	4 g
Iron	1 mg
Calcium	189 mg

- Blender

1/2	small banana	1/2
1 1/2 cups	strawberries	375 mL
1 cup	fortified GF non-dairy milk or lactose-free 1% milk (see tip, page 150)	250 mL
1/2 cup	GF soy yogurt or yogurt	125 mL
1 tbsp	ground flax seeds (flaxseed meal)	15 mL

1. In a blender, combine banana, strawberries, milk, yogurt and flax seeds; blend for 1 minute.

Variations

Try using a flavored yogurt.

If you prefer to use lower-sugar fruit, try kiwifruit, peaches, apricots, blueberries or blackberries.

Breads and Muffins

Banana Almond Bread

Theresa loves banana bread so much that she came up with a recipe to accommodate nutrition and taste. Alex suggested the addition of dried apricots and teff flour for more iron and fiber and almonds for extra calcium.

Tip

If you don't have a glass loaf dish, use a metal loaf pan and increase the baking time by 5 to 10 minutes.

- Preheat oven to 350°F (180°C)
- 9- by 5-inch (23 by 12.5 cm) glass loaf dish, greased, bottom lined with parchment paper

¾ cup	sorghum flour	175 mL
¼ cup	teff flour	60 mL
2 tsp	GF baking powder	10 mL
1 tsp	baking soda	5 mL
¼ tsp	salt	1 mL
2	eggs	2
½ cup	granulated raw cane sugar	125 mL
⅓ cup	vegetable oil	75 mL
1 tsp	almond extract	5 mL
1 cup	mashed ripe bananas	250 mL
¼ cup	chopped dried apricots	60 mL
¼ cup	slivered almonds	60 mL

1. In a large bowl, whisk together sorghum flour, teff flour, baking powder, baking soda and salt.

2. In a medium bowl, whisk together eggs, sugar, oil and almond extract until well blended. Stir in bananas. Pour over dry ingredients and stir until combined. Gently fold in apricots and almonds.

3. Pour batter into prepared loaf dish. Bake in preheated oven for about 50 minutes or until a tester inserted in the center comes out clean. Let cool in dish on a wire rack for 10 minutes. Remove from dish and peel off paper. Transfer loaf to rack and let cool completely.

Nutrients Per Serving	
Calories	260
Carbohydrate	34 g
Fiber	3 g
Protein	5 g
Fat	13 g
Iron	1 mg
Calcium	35 mg

Cranberry Banana Loaf

**Makes 8 slices
(1 slice per serving)**

This loaf was one of the first recipes Theresa's family learned to love when starting on a gluten-free diet, and it's always gone by the end of the day. The quinoa flour is a recent addition, for extra nutritional value.

Tip

There's no need to wait for the frozen cranberries to thaw; just add them to the batter straight from the freezer.

If you don't have a glass loaf dish, use a metal loaf pan and increase the baking time by 5 to 10 minutes.

- Preheat oven to 350°F (180°C)
- 9- by 5-inch (23 by 12.5 cm) glass loaf dish, greased, bottom lined with parchment paper

1/2 cup	white rice flour	125 mL
1/4 cup	brown rice flour	60 mL
1/4 cup	quinoa flour	60 mL
2 tsp	GF baking powder	10 mL
1 1/2 tsp	ground cinnamon	7 mL
1/4 tsp	salt	1 mL
1/2 cup	granulated raw cane sugar	125 mL
1/4 cup	butter or vegan hard margarine, softened	60 mL
2	eggs	2
1 cup	mashed ripe bananas	250 mL
1 cup	fresh or frozen cranberries	250 mL

1. In a medium bowl, whisk together white rice flour, brown rice flour, quinoa flour, baking powder, cinnamon and salt.

2. In a large bowl, using an electric mixer, cream sugar and butter until light and fluffy. Beat in eggs, one at a time, until well blended. Stir in bananas. Stir in dry ingredients until combined. Gently fold in cranberries.

3. Pour batter into prepared loaf dish. Bake in preheated oven for 45 to 50 minutes or until a tester inserted in the center comes out clean. Let cool in dish on a wire rack for 10 minutes. Remove from dish and peel off paper. Transfer loaf to rack and let cool completely.

Nutrients Per Serving	
Calories	210
Carbohydrate	33 g
Fiber	2 g
Protein	3 g
Fat	7 g
Iron	1 mg
Calcium	12 mg

Pear and Walnut Loaf

Apples are a common baking ingredient, but pears work just as well and make for a nice change.

Tip

Choose pears that feel hard when gently squeezed at the neck near the stem. Be sure not to use pears that are ripe and soft, as these will be too juicy for this loaf. Don't bother peeling the pears — the skin adds to the nutrition, texture and appearance of the loaf.

- Preheat oven to 350°F (180°C)
- 9- by 5-inch (23 by 12.5 cm) loaf pan, greased, bottom lined with parchment paper

1 cup	sorghum flour	250 mL
¼ cup	tapioca starch	60 mL
2 tsp	GF baking powder	10 mL
¼ tsp	salt	1 mL
¼ tsp	ground cinnamon	1 mL
½ cup	granulated raw cane sugar	125 mL
¼ cup	butter, softened	60 mL
2	eggs	2
1 tsp	vanilla extract	5 mL
1 cup	coarsely shredded firm pears (about 2)	250 mL
1 cup	chopped walnuts	250 mL

1. In a medium bowl, whisk together sorghum flour, tapioca starch, baking powder, salt and cinnamon.

2. In a large bowl, using an electric mixer, cream sugar and butter until light and fluffy. Beat in eggs, one at a time, until well blended. Stir in vanilla. Stir in dry ingredients until just combined. Gently fold in pears and walnuts.

3. Pour batter into prepared loaf dish. Bake in preheated oven for 50 to 60 minutes or until a tester inserted in the center comes out clean. Let cool in dish on a wire rack for 10 minutes. Remove from dish and peel off paper. Transfer loaf to rack and let cool completely.

Nutrients Per Serving	
Calories	280
Carbohydrate	34 g
Fiber	3 g
Protein	6 g
Fat	17 g
Iron	1 mg
Calcium	33 mg

Brown Sandwich Bread

This moist bread, which slices with ease, is perfect for sandwiches. Or enjoy it with butter and jam, as Theresa's husband does.

Tips

Warm the milk in a glass measuring cup in the microwave on High for about 1 minute, or the traditional way, in a small saucepan over low heat.

If you don't have a glass loaf dish, use a metal loaf pan and increase the baking time by 5 to 10 minutes.

Let bread cool completely before slicing. Use a serrated bread knife for the best results. Wrap cooled bread and store at room temperature for up to 4 days or freeze for up to 1 month.

Nutrients Per Serving

Calories	110
Carbohydrate	15 g
Fiber	2 g
Protein	3 g
Fat	4 g
Iron	0.5 mg
Calcium	23 mg

- Stand mixer
- 9- by 5-inch (23 by 12.5 cm) glass loaf dish, greased, bottom lined with parchment paper

1 cup	sorghum flour	250 mL
1/3 cup	psyllium husks	75 mL
1/4 cup	white rice flour	60 mL
1/4 cup	brown rice flour	60 mL
1/4 cup	tapioca starch	60 mL
2 tbsp	granulated raw cane sugar	30 mL
1 tsp	salt	5 mL
1/4 cup	cold butter, cut into cubes	60 mL
2 tsp	instant yeast	10 mL
1 cup	lactose-free 1% milk, heated to 120°F to 130°F (50°C to 55°C)	250 mL
2	eggs, lightly beaten	2

1. In large bowl of stand mixer, combine sorghum flour, psyllium, white rice flour, brown rice flour, tapioca starch, sugar, salt and butter. Beat on low speed until butter is incorporated. Add yeast and beat for 1 minute.

2. With motor running on low, gradually pour in heated milk, beating until incorporated. Beat for 1 minute. Beat in eggs until incorporated. Beat for 5 minutes, stopping mixer and scraping down sides of bowl and beater halfway through.

3. Spread batter in prepared loaf dish. Cover with a lint-free towel and let rise in a warm, draft-free place for 1 hour or until doubled in bulk. Meanwhile, preheat oven to 350°F (180°C).

4. Bake for 35 to 40 minutes or until browned and a tester inserted in the center comes out clean. Let cool in dish on a wire rack for 5 minutes. Run a knife around edge of bread and remove from dish. Peel off paper, transfer bread to rack and let cool completely.

Olive and Herb Flatbread

This delicious bread can accompany lunch or dinner or can be served as a dipping bread for appetizers.

Tips

Warm the milk in a glass measuring cup in the microwave on High for about 1 minute or the traditional way, in a small saucepan over low heat.

Two tbsp (30 mL) olive oil mixed with 1 tsp (5 mL) GF vinegar makes a nice dip for this flatbread.

Nutrients Per Serving

Calories	220
Carbohydrate	30 g
Fiber	5 g
Protein	6 g
Fat	9 g
Iron	1 mg
Calcium	52 mg

- Stand mixer
- 8-inch (23 cm) square glass baking dish, lightly greased with olive oil, bottom lined with parchment paper

1 cup	sorghum flour	250 mL
1/3 cup	psyllium husks	75 mL
1/4 cup	white rice flour	60 mL
1/4 cup	brown rice flour	60 mL
1/4 cup	tapioca starch	60 mL
2 tbsp	granulated raw cane sugar	30 mL
1 tbsp	dried Italian seasoning	15 mL
1 tsp	salt	5 mL
1/4 cup	cold butter, cut into cubes	60 mL
2 tsp	instant yeast	10 mL
1 cup	lactose-free 1% milk, heated to 120°F to 130°F (50°C to 55°C)	250 mL
2	eggs, lightly beaten	2
1/2 cup	sliced kalamata olives	125 mL

Topping

1 tsp	olive oil	5 mL
	Dried Italian seasoning	
	Salt and freshly ground black pepper	

1. In large bowl of stand mixer, combine sorghum flour, psyllium, white rice flour, brown rice flour, tapioca starch, sugar, Italian seasoning, salt and butter. Beat on low speed until butter is incorporated. Add yeast and beat for 1 minute.

2. With motor running on low, gradually pour in heated milk, beating until incorporated. Beat for 1 minute. Beat in eggs until incorporated. Beat for 5 minutes, stopping mixer and scraping down sides of bowl and beater halfway through. Beat in olives until incorporated. Spread batter in prepared baking dish.

3. *Topping:* Brush dough with olive oil and season to taste with Italian seasoning, salt and pepper. Cover with a lint-free towel and let rise in a warm, draft-free place for 1 hour or until doubled in bulk. Meanwhile, preheat oven to 350°F (180°C).

4. Bake for 35 to 40 minutes or until browned and a tester inserted in the center comes out clean. Let cool in dish on a wire rack for 5 minutes. Run a knife around edge of bread and remove from dish. Peel off paper, transfer bread to rack and let cool completely.

Popovers

Makes 12 popovers (1 per serving)

These are an absolute treat alongside any soup or with a roast beef meal. They're the next best thing to Yorkshire pudding.

Tip

Choose your favorite GF non-dairy milk, such as soy, rice, almond or potato-based milk or, if you tolerate lactose, use regular 1% milk.

- Preheat oven to 450°F (230°C)
- 12-cup muffin pan, greased

½ cup	white rice flour	125 mL
1 tbsp	psyllium husks	15 mL
¼ tsp	salt	1 mL
2	eggs, lightly beaten	2
1 cup	lactose-free 1% milk or fortified GF non-dairy milk	250 mL
1 tbsp	melted butter	15 mL

1. In a large bowl, combine white rice flour, psyllium husks and salt.

2. In another bowl, whisk together eggs, milk and butter. Pour into dry ingredients and stir until smooth.

3. Pour batter into prepared muffin cups, dividing equally. Bake in preheated oven for 15 minutes. Reduce heat to 350°F (180°C) and bake for 5 minutes or until golden brown. Let cool in pan on a wire rack for 5 minutes. Run a knife around edge of pan to loosen popovers. Serve hot.

Psyllium Husks

Psyllium husks are the outer part of psyllium seeds, which are from the plantain plant, *Plantago ovato*. Numerous large-scale studies have shown that daily consumption of small amounts of psyllium fiber (3 to 12 grams a day) can help reduce LDL cholesterol ("bad" cholesterol). Other research indicates that when psyllium is incorporated into food, it is more effective at reducing the blood glucose response than a soluble fiber supplement that is taken separately from food.

Nutrients Per Serving

Calories	50
Carbohydrate	6 g
Fiber	1 g
Protein	2 g
Fat	2 g
Iron	0.2 mg
Calcium	33 mg

Traditional Tea Biscuits

Makes 12 biscuits (1 per serving)

One of the things Theresa really used to miss on the gluten-free diet was tea biscuits, but not anymore! She serves these up with butter and jam.

Tip

Choose your favorite GF non-dairy milk, such as soy, rice, almond or potato-based milk or, if you tolerate lactose, use regular 1% milk.

Variation

Traditional Tea Biscuits with Raisins: Add ½ tsp (2 mL) ground cinnamon with the baking powder and add ½ cup (125 mL) raisins to the dough at the end of step 2. Bake as directed.

- Preheat oven to 350°F (180°C)
- Baking sheet, lined with parchment paper

½ cup	potato starch	125 mL
¼ cup	sorghum flour	60 mL
¼ cup	brown rice flour	60 mL
1 tbsp	granulated raw cane sugar	15 mL
2 tsp	GF baking powder	10 mL
2 tbsp	cold butter or vegan hard margarine, cut into pieces	30 mL
1	egg white, lightly beaten	1
¼ cup	lactose-free 1% milk or fortified GF non-dairy milk	60 mL

1. In a large bowl, combine potato starch, sorghum flour, brown rice flour, sugar and baking powder. Using a pastry blender or two knives, cut in butter until mixture resembles coarse crumbs about the size of small peas.

2. In another bowl, whisk together egg white and milk. Pour into dry ingredients and stir until just combined.

3. Using a spoon, scoop out 12 spoonfuls of dough and place about 2 inches (5 cm) apart on prepared baking sheet. Bake in preheated oven for 10 to 12 minutes or until firm to the touch. Let cool on pan on a wire rack for 5 minutes. Transfer biscuits to rack to cool slightly. Serve warm.

Nutrients Per Serving

Calories	70
Carbohydrate	13 g
Fiber	0 g
Protein	1 g
Fat	2 g
Iron	0.2 mg
Calcium	14 mg

Savory Tea Biscuits

These tea biscuits are a great accompaniment to any meat or soup dish.

Tip

Choose your favorite GF non-dairy milk, such as soy, rice, almond or potato-based milk or, if you tolerate lactose, use 1% milk.

- Preheat oven to 350°F (180°C)
- Baking sheet, lined with parchment paper

½ cup	potato starch	125 mL
¼ cup	sorghum flour	60 mL
¼ cup	brown rice flour	60 mL
1 tbsp	granulated raw cane sugar	15 mL
2 tsp	GF baking powder	10 mL
2 tbsp	cold hard vegan margarine or butter, cut into pieces	30 mL
1	egg white, lightly beaten	1
¼ cup	lactose-free 1% milk or fortified GF non-dairy milk	60 mL
¼ cup	diced drained oil-packed sun-dried tomatoes	60 mL
¼ cup	grated Romano cheese	60 mL
½ tsp	paprika	2 mL
½ tsp	dried Italian seasoning	2 mL

1. In a large bowl, combine potato starch, sorghum flour, brown rice flour, sugar and baking powder. Using a pastry blender or two knives, cut in margarine until mixture resembles coarse crumbs about the size of small peas.

2. In another bowl, whisk together egg white and milk. Pour into dry ingredients and stir until just combined. Stir in tomatoes, cheese, paprika and Italian seasoning.

3. Using a spoon, scoop out 15 spoonfuls of dough and place about 2 inches (5 cm) apart on prepared baking sheet. Bake in preheated oven for 10 to 12 minutes or until tops are golden. Let cool on pan on a wire rack for 5 minutes. Transfer biscuits to rack to cool slightly. Serve warm.

Nutrients Per Serving	
Calories	90
Carbohydrate	13 g
Fiber	1 g
Protein	2 g
Fat	4 g
Iron	0.3 mg
Calcium	43 mg

Millet and Flax Muffins

When Theresa says the words "healthy muffins," her sons cringe. But when muffins have great flavor, as these ones do, it's easy to forget they're a healthier alternative. Serve these to accompany any chicken dish when you want to wow your friends.

Tip

Choose your favorite GF non-dairy milk, such as soy, rice, almond or potato-based milk or, if you tolerate lactose, use regular 1% milk.

- Preheat oven to 350°F (180°C)
- 12-cup muffin pan, 9 cups lined with paper liners

1/2 cup	millet grits	125 mL
1/4 cup	brown rice flour	60 mL
1/4 cup	ground flax seeds (flaxseed meal)	60 mL
2 tsp	GF baking powder	10 mL
1	egg	1
2 tbsp	granulated raw cane sugar	30 mL
1/2 cup	lactose-free 1% milk or fortified GF non-dairy milk	125 mL
2 tbsp	unsweetened applesauce	30 mL

1. In a large bowl, whisk together millet grits, brown rice flour, flax seeds and baking powder.

2. In a medium bowl, whisk together egg, sugar, milk and applesauce until well combined. Pour over dry ingredients and stir until combined.

3. Spoon batter into prepared muffin cups, dividing equally. Bake in preheated oven for 15 to 20 minutes or until a tester inserted in the center comes out clean. Let cool in pan on a wire rack for 5 minutes. Transfer muffins to rack to cool.

Nutrients Per Serving	
Calories	100
Carbohydrate	18 g
Fiber	3 g
Protein	4 g
Fat	3 g
Iron	2 mg
Calcium	33 mg

Apricot Oatmeal Muffins

When introducing pure, uncontaminated oats into your diet, begin with small amounts, such as one of these muffins at breakfast time. For more information, see page 43.

Tip

Make sure the oats you buy are labeled "pure oats" or have a gluten-free certification — this assures you that there has been no cross-contamination with wheat, barley or rye.

Choose your favorite GF non-dairy milk, such as soy, rice, almond or potato-based milk or, if you tolerate lactose, use regular 1% milk.

- Preheat oven to 350°F (180°C)
- 12-cup muffin pan, lined with paper liners

½ cup	sorghum flour	125 mL
½ cup	tapioca starch	125 mL
½ cup	GF large-flake (old-fashioned) rolled oats	125 mL
2 tsp	GF baking powder	10 mL
1 tsp	ground cinnamon	5 mL
2	eggs	2
¼ cup	granulated raw cane sugar	60 mL
½ cup	fortified GF non-dairy milk or lactose-free 1% milk	125 mL
¼ cup	sunflower oil	60 mL
¼ cup	light (fancy) molasses	60 mL
½ cup	chopped apricots	125 mL
½ cup	chopped walnuts	125 mL

1. In a large bowl, whisk together sorghum flour, tapioca starch, oats, baking powder and cinnamon.

2. In a medium bowl, whisk together eggs, sugar, milk, oil and molasses until well combined. Pour over dry ingredients and stir until combined. Gently fold in apricots and walnuts.

3. Spoon batter into prepared muffin cups, dividing equally. Bake in preheated oven for about 25 minutes or until a tester inserted in the center comes out clean. Let cool in pan on a wire rack for 5 minutes. Transfer muffins to rack to cool.

Nutrients Per Serving

Calories	200
Carbohydrate	27 g
Fiber	2 g
Protein	5 g
Fat	10 g
Iron	2 mg
Calcium	57 mg

Yummy Doodle Muffins

Remember the scene in the movie *The Holiday* where Jack Black sings a little ditty at the piano with Kate Winslet? It goes like this: "Yummily, doodley do do..." Theresa was thinking of this song when she named these muffins, because they are so yummily, doodley delicious!

- Preheat oven to 350°F (180°C)
- 12-cup muffin pan, lined with paper liners

½ cup	millet grits	125 mL
½ cup	brown rice flour	125 mL
¼ cup	potato starch	60 mL
2 tsp	GF baking powder	10 mL
1 tsp	ground cinnamon	5 mL
2	eggs	2
¼ cup	granulated raw cane sugar	60 mL
1 cup	unsweetened applesauce	250 mL
2 tbsp	grapeseed oil	30 mL
1 tsp	vanilla extract	5 mL
1 cup	chopped walnuts	250 mL
1 cup	sliced dried apricots or chopped dried cherries	250 mL

1. In a large bowl, whisk together millet grits, brown rice flour, potato starch, baking powder and cinnamon.

2. In a medium bowl, whisk together eggs, sugar, applesauce, oil and vanilla until well combined. Pour over dry ingredients and stir until combined. Gently fold in walnuts and apricots.

3. Spoon batter into prepared muffin cups, dividing equally. Bake in preheated oven for 20 to 25 minutes or until a tester inserted in the center comes out clean. Let cool in pan on a wire rack for 5 minutes. Transfer muffins to rack to cool.

Nutrients Per Serving	
Calories	220
Carbohydrate	31 g
Fiber	3 g
Protein	4 g
Fat	10 g
Iron	2 mg
Calcium	29 mg

Chunky Blueberry Muffins

These muffins freeze well, so you can always have them on hand for a quick breakfast or snack. Just microwave one for 20 seconds and you're good to go.

Tips

To easily zest a lemon, use a rasp grater, such as a Microplane.

Choose your favorite GF non-dairy milk, such as soy, rice, almond or potato-based milk or, if you tolerate lactose, use regular 1% milk.

- Preheat oven to 350°F (180°C)
- 12-cup muffin pan, lined with paper liners

½ cup	brown rice flour	125 mL
¼ cup	sorghum flour	60 mL
¼ cup	potato starch	60 mL
¼ cup	ground flax seeds (flaxseed meal)	60 mL
2 tsp	GF baking powder	10 mL
½ tsp	salt	2 mL
2	eggs	2
¼ cup	granulated raw cane sugar	60 mL
½ cup	unsweetened applesauce	125 mL
¼ cup	fortified GF non-dairy milk or lactose-free 1% milk	60 mL
1 cup	chopped peeled apples	250 mL
1 cup	fresh or frozen blueberries	250 mL
¼ cup	chopped walnuts	60 mL
2 tsp	grated lemon zest	10 mL

1. In a large bowl, whisk together brown rice flour, sorghum flour, potato starch, flax seeds, baking powder and salt.

2. In a medium bowl, whisk together eggs, sugar, applesauce and milk until well combined. Pour over dry ingredients and stir until combined. Gently fold in apples, blueberries, walnuts and lemon zest.

3. Spoon batter into prepared muffin cups, dividing equally. Bake in preheated oven for 20 to 25 minutes or until a tester inserted in the center comes out clean. Let cool in pan on a wire rack for 5 minutes. Transfer muffins to rack to cool.

Nutrients Per Serving	
Calories	120
Carbohydrate	20 g
Fiber	2 g
Protein	3 g
Fat	3.5 g
Iron	1 mg
Calcium	26 mg

Pineapple Carrot Muffins

This recipe is low in fat and high in flavor and nutrients — a win-win!

Tip

To toast walnuts, spread chopped nuts on a baking sheet and bake in a 350°F (180°C) oven for 5 to 8 minutes, or toast in a dry skillet over medium heat, stirring constantly, for 3 to 5 minutes, until toasted and fragrant.

- Preheat oven to 350°F (180°C)
- 12-cup muffin pan, lined with paper liners

1/2 cup	brown rice flour	125 mL
1/4 cup	sorghum flour	60 mL
1/4 cup	teff flour	60 mL
2 tsp	GF baking powder	10 mL
1 tsp	ground cinnamon	5 mL
1/4 tsp	salt	1 mL
2	eggs	2
1/4 cup	granulated raw cane sugar	60 mL
1 tbsp	vegetable oil	15 mL
1 cup	canned unsweetened crushed pineapple	250 mL
1 cup	shredded carrots	250 mL
1/2 cup	chopped walnuts, toasted	125 mL

1. In a large bowl, whisk together brown rice flour, sorghum flour, teff flour, baking powder, cinnamon and salt.

2. In a medium bowl, whisk together eggs, sugar and oil until well combined. Stir in pineapple. Pour over dry ingredients and stir until combined. Gently fold in carrots and walnuts.

3. Spoon batter into prepared muffin cups, dividing equally. Bake in preheated oven for 25 to 30 minutes or until a tester inserted in the center comes out clean. Let cool in pan on a wire rack for 5 minutes. Transfer muffins to rack to cool.

Nutrients Per Serving	
Calories	130
Carbohydrate	18 g
Fiber	2 g
Protein	3 g
Fat	5 g
Iron	1 mg
Calcium	20 mg

Strawberry Almond Muffins

These fruity, nutty muffins
are great for a morning
snack or breakfast on
the go.

Tip
Choose your favorite
GF non-dairy milk, such
as soy, rice, almond or
potato-based milk or, if
you tolerate lactose, use
regular 1% milk.

- Preheat oven to 350°F (180°C)
- 12-cup muffin pan, 10 cups lined with paper liners

1/2 cup	sorghum flour	125 mL
1/2 cup	amaranth flour	125 mL
2 tsp	GF baking powder	10 mL
1/2 tsp	ground cinnamon	2 mL
1/4 tsp	salt	1 mL
1/2 cup	granulated raw cane sugar	125 mL
1/4 cup	butter or hard vegan margarine, softened	60 mL
1/4 cup	cream cheese or soy cream cheese alternative, softened	60 mL
1	egg	1
1/4 cup	lactose-free 1% milk or fortified GF non-dairy milk	60 mL
1 cup	chopped strawberries	250 mL
1 cup	slivered almonds	250 mL

1. In a medium bowl, combine sorghum flour, amaranth flour, baking powder, cinnamon and salt.

2. In a large bowl, using an electric mixer, cream sugar, butter and cream cheese. Beat in egg until well combined. Beat in milk. Stir in dry ingredients until just combined. Gently fold in strawberries and almonds.

3. Spoon batter into prepared muffin cups, dividing equally. Bake in preheated oven for 20 to 25 minutes or until a tester inserted in the center comes out clean. Let cool in pan on a wire rack for 5 minutes. Transfer muffins to rack to cool.

Nutrients Per Serving	
Calories	230
Carbohydrate	23 g
Fiber	3 g
Protein	6 g
Fat	14 g
Iron	1 mg
Calcium	68 mg

Zucchini Oatmeal Muffins

These muffins are low in
fat but big in flavor. While
they're baking, a delectable
aroma will waft through
your home — be patient
and let them cool a bit
before gobbling them up!

Tip

Leave the skin on the
zucchini — it adds nutrition
and color. If, however, your
children are anything like
Theresa's and you want
them to eat this tasty muffin
without detecting green
bits, you can peel off skin
before shredding.

- Preheat oven to 350°F (180°C)
- 12-cup muffin pan, lined with paper liners

½ cup	sorghum flour	125 mL
½ cup	GF large-flake (old-fashioned) rolled oats (see tip, page 163)	125 mL
¼ cup	raw unsalted sunflower seeds	60 mL
2 tsp	GF baking powder	10 mL
2 tsp	ground cinnamon	10 mL
2	eggs	2
¼ cup	granulated raw cane sugar	60 mL
¼ cup	unsweetened applesauce	60 mL
2 tbsp	grapeseed oil	30 mL
2 cups	shredded zucchini	500 mL
¼ cup	raisins	60 mL

1. In a large bowl, whisk together sorghum flour, oats, sunflower seeds, baking powder and cinnamon.

2. In a medium bowl, whisk together eggs, sugar, applesauce and oil until well combined. Stir in zucchini. Pour over dry ingredients and stir until combined. Gently fold in raisins.

3. Spoon batter into prepared muffin cups, dividing equally. Bake in preheated oven for 25 to 30 minutes or until a tester inserted in the center comes out clean. Let cool in pan on a wire rack for 5 minutes. Transfer muffins to rack to cool.

Nutrients Per Serving	
Calories	110
Carbohydrate	16 g
Fiber	2 g
Protein	3 g
Fat	5 g
Iron	1 mg
Calcium	25 mg

Soups and Salads

Turkey Broth

This versatile broth can be made whenever you cook a whole turkey. Store the carcass in a large pot in the refrigerator, then make broth the next day. Some of the broth can be immediately turned into Quinoa Soup (see box), the rest stored in the freezer.

Tip

Once the broth has cooled, divide it into 1- to 2-cup (250 to 500 mL) portions and store in airtight containers in the freezer for up to 1 month.

Variation

A chicken carcass, or uncooked turkey or chicken pieces and bones, can be substituted for the turkey carcass. Make sure to save any good meat when straining the broth.

Nutrients Per Serving	
Calories	20
Carbohydrate	0 g
Fiber	0 g
Protein	2 g
Fat	1 g
Iron	0 mg
Calcium	0 mg

1	turkey carcass	1
1 tsp	salt	5 mL
1	carrot	1
1	stalk celery	1
1	onion, peeled	1
3 tbsp	tomato sauce	45 mL

1. Place turkey carcass in a large pot. Cover with 12 cups (3 L) water and sprinkle with salt. Bring to a boil over medium-high heat.

2. When scum forms on the surface, skim it off. Stir in carrot, celery, onion and tomato sauce. Cover, leaving lid ajar, reduce heat to low and simmer for $1\frac{1}{2}$ hours.

3. Gradually ladle broth into a fine-mesh strainer set over another large pot, pressing solids to press out as much liquid as possible. Discard solids.

Quinoa Soup

To easily turn this broth into a hearty soup that serves 2 people, bring 2 cups (500 mL) broth to a boil, then stir in $\frac{1}{4}$ cup (60 mL) quinoa, rinsed, or long-grain rice. Reduce heat to low, cover and simmer for 20 minutes or until quinoa is tender.

(Nutrients Per Serving: Calories: 90; Carbohydrate: 15 g; Fiber: 1 g; Protein: 4 g; Fat: 1.5 g; Iron: 1 mg; Calcium: 10 mg)

To make it even heartier, try adding chopped carrots, chopped celery and chunks of cooked chicken or turkey with the quinoa.

Minestrone

Makes 6 to 8 servings

Theresa's mom graciously agreed to share this simple, delicious recipe with you. The ingredients for minestrone can change from week to week, depending on what you have in the refrigerator. Be adventurous and try out whatever vegetables you have on hand — you won't be disappointed.

Tip

A 19-oz (540 mL) can of beans will yield about 2 cups (500 mL) once the beans are drained and rinsed. If you have smaller or larger cans, you can use the volume called for or just add the amount from your can.

Variations

Substitute cooked beef for the chicken.

Add 1 cup (250 mL) cooked GF pasta to the finished minestrone.

Nutrients Per Serving	
Calories	160
Carbohydrate	21 g
Fiber	5 g
Protein	11 g
Fat	4 g
Iron	2 mg
Calcium	43 mg

1 tbsp	grapeseed oil	15 mL
1	clove garlic, minced	1
1/2 cup	chopped onion	125 mL
1 tbsp	chopped fresh parsley	15 mL
1	potato (unpeeled), chopped	1
1	tomato, chopped	1
2 cups	rinsed drained canned romano beans	500 mL
1 cup	cubed cooked chicken	250 mL
1/2 cup	peas	125 mL
1/2 cup	broccoli florets	125 mL
1/2 cup	chopped celery	125 mL
1/4 cup	chopped dry-packed sun-dried tomatoes	60 mL
	Salt and freshly ground black pepper	

1. In a large saucepan, heat oil over medium heat. Sauté garlic, onion and parsley for 3 to 4 minutes or until onion is softened.

2. Stir in potato, chopped tomato, beans, chicken, peas, broccoli, celery, sun-dried tomatoes and 8 cups (2 L) water; bring to a boil over medium-high heat. Cover, leaving lid ajar, reduce heat to low and simmer, stirring occasionally, for 30 minutes or until vegetables are tender (or for up to 1 1/2 hours if you prefer a very soft texture). Season to taste with salt and pepper.

Potato, Leek and Broccoli Soup

Makes 6 to
8 servings

This yummy soup can be
either chunky or smooth,
depending on how your
family likes it.

Tips

Leeks hold a lot of dirt in
their layers and must be
rinsed thoroughly under
cold running water before
they are sliced.

If you have an immersion
blender, you can purée
the soup right in the pot.

2 tbsp	grapeseed oil	30 mL
2	leeks (white and light green parts only), sliced	2
4 cups	reduced-sodium GF vegetable broth	1 L
2	potatoes, peeled and chopped	2
2 cups	chopped fresh or frozen broccoli	500 mL
1 tsp	salt	5 mL
¼ tsp	freshly ground black pepper	1 mL

1. In a large pot, heat oil over medium-high heat. Sauté leeks for 4 to 5 minutes or until wilted. Add broth and 4 cups (1 L) water; bring to a boil. Add potatoes, broccoli, salt and pepper; return to a boil. Reduce heat and simmer for 15 minutes or until potatoes are tender.

2. Serve chunky or, to serve smooth, transfer soup in batches to a food processor or blender and purée to desired consistency.

Nutrients Per Serving

Calories	90
Carbohydrate	13 g
Fiber	3 g
Protein	2 g
Fat	3 g
Iron	1 mg
Calcium	47 mg

Winter Soup Purée

This recipe comes to you courtesy of Theresa's friend Dawn-Angela. It's wonderful served with Popovers (page 159).

Tip

To cut down the prep time, purchase precut vegetables.

4 cups	reduced-sodium GF chicken broth	1 L
2 cups	chopped onions	500 mL
2 cups	chopped parsnips	500 mL
2 cups	chopped carrots	500 mL
2 cups	chopped broccoli	500 mL
1 cup	chopped turnip	250 mL
5	bay leaves	5
	Ground nutmeg	
	Salt and freshly ground black pepper	

1. In a large pot, combine broth, 4 cups (1 L) water, onions, parsnips, carrots, broccoli, turnip, bay leaves and a pinch of nutmeg. Bring to a boil over medium-high heat. Cover, reduce heat to low and simmer, stirring occasionally, for 45 to 60 minutes or until vegetables are tender. Discard bay leaves.

2. Using an immersion blender, or in batches in a food processor or blender, purée soup until smooth. Season to taste with salt and pepper. Serve sprinkled with nutmeg.

Nutrients Per Serving

Calories	80
Carbohydrate	16 g
Fiber	4 g
Protein	3 g
Fat	0 g
Iron	1 mg
Calcium	50 mg

Soup à la Mom

Theresa's mom never seemed to measure anything when making soup; she just threw in a handful of this, a little of that. But to help you achieve her magnificent results, Theresa has done the measuring for you. It takes awhile to chop all the vegetables, but it's so worth it in the end.

Tips

The longer this soup simmers, the better it tastes.

This soup freezes well. Let cool, divide into individual portions and freeze in airtight containers for up to 1 month.

2 tbsp	grapeseed oil	30 mL
3	green onions, chopped	3
3 tbsp	chopped fresh parsley	45 mL
2	carrots, chopped	2
2	stalks celery, chopped	2
1	zucchini, chopped	1
2 cups	rinsed drained canned chickpeas (see tip, page 171)	500 mL
2 cups	frozen peas	500 mL
2 cups	frozen chopped green beans	500 mL
2 cups	frozen lima or butter beans	500 mL
4 cups	reduced-sodium GF chicken broth	1 L
1/4 cup	tomato sauce (or 1 tomato, chopped)	60 mL
1/4 tsp	salt	1 mL
1/4 tsp	freshly ground black pepper	1 mL

1. In a large pot, heat oil over medium heat. Sauté green onions and parsley for about 3 minutes or until onions are softened.

2. Stir in carrots, celery, zucchini, chickpeas, peas, green beans, lima beans, broth, 4 cups (1 L) water, tomato sauce, salt and pepper. Cover, leaving lid ajar, reduce heat to low and simmer, stirring occasionally, for 30 minutes or until vegetables are tender (or for up to 1 hour if you prefer a very soft texture).

Nutrients Per Serving	
Calories	160
Carbohydrate	25 g
Fiber	7 g
Protein	8 g
Fat	0 g
Iron	2 mg
Calcium	56 mg

Lentil and Spinach Soup

Makes 4 servings

Theresa's son Eli is a soup hound. One night he came home from a friend's house raving about her lentil soup. She was kind enough to share it with Theresa, and with you.

Tip

Look for bags of spinach that have been frozen in small cubes rather than in a large block. You can measure the cubes and add them to the pot without thawing them. If you can't find them, use ½ cup (125 mL) drained thawed chopped spinach.

2 tbsp	olive oil	30 mL
2	cloves garlic, minced	2
¼ cup	chopped onion	60 mL
¼ cup	chopped celery	60 mL
½ cup	chopped carrots	125 mL
2 cups	rinsed drained canned lentils (see tip, page 171)	500 mL
1 cup	frozen spinach cubes	250 mL
4 cups	Turkey Broth (see recipe, page 170) or reduced-sodium GF chicken or vegetable broth	1 L
	Salt and freshly ground black pepper	

1. In a large saucepan, heat oil over medium heat. Sauté garlic, onion, celery and carrots for 3 to 4 minutes or until softened.

2. Stir in lentils, spinach and broth; bring to a boil over high heat. Cover, leaving lid ajar, reduce heat to low and simmer, stirring occasionally, for 30 minutes or until vegetables are tender (or for up to 1 hour if you prefer a very soft texture). Season to taste with salt and pepper.

Nutrients Per Serving

Calories	220
Carbohydrate	26 g
Fiber	10 g
Protein	13 g
Fat	8 g
Iron	5 mg
Calcium	81 mg

Chickpea Soup

Makes 6 to 8 servings

Theresa's mom is the genius behind this simple recipe, which is a great accompaniment to any meal.

Tip

A 19-oz (540 mL) can of chickpeas will yield about 2 cups (500 mL) once the beans are drained and rinsed. If you have smaller or larger cans, you can use the volume called for or just add the amount from your can.

8	small potatoes, cut into bite-size pieces	8
4 cups	reduced-sodium GF vegetable or chicken broth	1 L
2 cups	rinsed drained canned chickpeas	500 mL
½ tsp	dried rosemary	2 mL

1. In a large pot, combine potatoes, broth, chickpeas, rosemary and 4 cups (1 L) water. Bring to a boil over medium-high heat. Cover, leaving lid ajar, reduce heat to low and simmer, stirring occasionally, for 30 minutes or until potatoes are tender (or for up to 1 hour if you prefer a very soft texture).

Nutrients Per Serving

Calories	190
Carbohydrate	40 g
Fiber	6 g
Protein	6 g
Fat	1 g
Iron	2 mg
Calcium	41 mg

Pasta e Fagioli

This traditional Italian soup of pasta and beans was a staple in Theresa's house when she was growing up. This version uses gluten-free pasta.

Tips

A 19-oz (540 mL) can of beans will yield about 2 cups (500 mL) once the beans are drained and rinsed. If you have smaller or larger cans, you can use the volume called for or just add the amount from your can.

You can use your favorite variety and shape of GF pasta in this soup. Look for new, extra-nutritious varieties such as a quinoa and brown rice blend.

1 tbsp	grapeseed oil	15 mL
1	clove garlic, minced	1
½ cup	chopped onion	125 mL
1 tbsp	chopped fresh parsley	15 mL
4 cups	reduced-sodium GF vegetable or chicken broth	1 L
2 cups	rinsed drained canned romano beans	500 mL
3 tbsp	tomato sauce	45 mL
8 oz	GF short pasta (see tip, at left)	250 g
	Salt (optional)	
¼ cup	grated Romano cheese	60 mL

1. In a large saucepan, heat oil over medium heat. Sauté garlic, onion and parsley for 3 to 4 minutes or until onion is softened.

2. Stir in broth, beans and tomato sauce; bring to a boil. Reduce heat and simmer, stirring occasionally, for 35 to 45 minutes to blend the flavors.

3. Meanwhile, in a large pot of boiling water, cook pasta according to package instructions until tender but firm (al dente). Drain.

4. Stir pasta into soup and season to taste with salt, if desired. Serve sprinkled with cheese.

Nutrients Per Serving	
Calories	440
Carbohydrate	77 g
Fiber	12 g
Protein	17 g
Fat	7 g
Iron	6 mg
Calcium	199 mg

Cranberry Mandarin Coleslaw with Walnuts and Raisins

This yummy salad is perfect for backyard barbecues and summer picnics — or anytime you host a large gathering of family and friends. It is made the night before the party, so it's a great time-saver the day of the event.

3 cups	shredded red and/or green cabbage	750 mL
2 cups	shredded carrots	500 mL
1 cup	chopped celery	250 mL
½ cup	chopped green onions	125 mL
1 tbsp	freshly squeezed lemon juice	15 mL
½ cup	raisins	125 mL
½ cup	raw green pumpkin seeds (pepitas)	125 mL
½ cup	fresh cranberries	125 mL
½ cup	walnut halves	125 mL
6 tbsp	extra virgin olive oil	90 mL
¼ cup	brown or natural rice vinegar	60 mL
1	can (10 oz/284 mL) mandarin oranges, drained	1

1. In a large bowl, combine cabbage, carrots, celery and green onions. Drizzle with lemon juice and toss to coat. Toss in raisins, pumpkin seeds, cranberries and walnuts.

2. In a small bowl, whisk together oil and vinegar. Drizzle over salad and toss to coat. Top with mandarin oranges. Cover and refrigerate overnight to blend the flavors.

Nutrients Per Serving

Calories	230
Carbohydrate	19 g
Fiber	3 g
Protein	4 g
Fat	16 g
Iron	2 mg
Calcium	34 mg

Everyday Salad

Makes 4 servings

When Theresa was growing up, salad was served with each evening meal. With its bright colors and fresh flavors, this is a terrific salad for every day.

Tip

For the dried herbs, Theresa loves the dried Italian seasoning blend. You can also use basil or thyme, or a combination.

4 cups	packed baby spinach leaves (about 6 oz/175 g)	1 L
½ cup	shredded red cabbage	125 mL
½ cup	sliced peeled cucumber	125 mL
½ cup	chopped yellow bell pepper	125 mL
¼ cup	chopped red bell pepper	60 mL
20	cherry tomatoes	20
2 tbsp	balsamic vinegar	30 mL
1½ tbsp	extra virgin olive oil	22 mL
1 tsp	dried herbs (see tip, at left)	5 mL
	Salt and freshly ground black pepper	

1. In a large bowl, combine spinach, cabbage, cucumber, yellow pepper, red pepper and tomatoes.

2. In a small bowl, whisk together vinegar, oil and herbs. Drizzle over salad and toss to coat. Season to taste with salt and pepper.

Nutrients Per Serving	
Calories	90
Carbohydrate	9 g
Fiber	2 g
Protein	2 g
Fat	6 g
Iron	1 mg
Calcium	43 mg

Greek Salad

Makes 4 servings

Theresa and Alex both love Greek salad, so they came up with this one to please the masses.

Nutrients Per Serving

Calories	200
Carbohydrate	13 g
Fiber	2 g
Protein	8 g
Fat	14 g
Iron	1 mg
Calcium	92 mg

2	tomatoes, cut into wedges	2
1	green bell pepper, chopped	1
2 cups	sliced English cucumber	500 mL
½ cup	sliced kalamata olives	125 mL
¼ cup	chopped red onion	60 mL
2 tbsp	extra virgin olive oil	30 mL
2 tbsp	brown or natural rice vinegar	30 mL
½ tsp	dried oregano	2 mL
	Salt and freshly ground black pepper	
½ cup	crumbled light or regular feta cheese	125 mL

1. In a large bowl, combine tomatoes, green pepper, cucumber, olives and onion.

2. In a small bowl, combine oil, vinegar and oregano. Drizzle over salad and toss to coat. Season to taste with salt and pepper. Sprinkle with feta cheese.

Orange and Olive Salad

Makes 4 servings

This simple yet delicious salad was a Christmas tradition in Theresa's mother's household in Italy. The only type of orange that grows in Italy is the blood orange, so that's the traditional choice, but any type of orange can be used.

Nutrients Per Serving

Calories	170
Carbohydrate	12 g
Fiber	3 g
Protein	1 g
Fat	13 g
Iron	2 mg
Calcium	76 mg

3	oranges, cut into bite-size pieces	3
1¾ cups	pitted black olives	425 mL
2 tbsp	extra virgin olive oil	30 mL
	Salt and freshly ground black pepper	

1. In a medium bowl, combine oranges and olives. Drizzle with olive oil and toss to coat. Season to taste with salt and pepper.

Chickpea Salad

Makes 6 to 8 servings

This is an excellent take-along salad for the beach or a picnic. It also makes a delicious, healthy snack when you get peckish. Theresa's family loves it all year long.

Tip

A 19-oz (540 mL) can of chickpeas will yield about 2 cups (500 mL) once the beans are drained and rinsed, so you'll need 2 cans of that size for this recipe. If you have smaller or larger cans, you can use the volume called for or just add the amount from your can.

4 cups	drained rinsed canned chickpeas	1 L
½ cup	chopped onion	125 mL
½ cup	chopped red bell pepper	125 mL
8	cherry tomatoes, quartered	8
2	cloves garlic, minced	2
2	carrots, chopped	2
3 tbsp	freshly squeezed lemon juice	45 mL
3 tbsp	rosemary-flavored vinegar	45 mL
2 tbsp	extra virgin olive oil	30 mL
1 tbsp	GF prepared mustard	15 mL
1 tsp	dried parsley	5 mL
1 tsp	dried basil	5 mL
½ tsp	dried oregano	2 mL
½ tsp	dried rosemary	2 mL
	Salt and freshly ground black pepper	

1. In a large bowl, combine chickpeas, onion, red pepper, tomatoes, garlic and carrots.

2. In a small bowl, whisk together lemon juice, vinegar, oil, mustard, parsley, basil, oregano and rosemary. Drizzle over salad and toss to coat. Season to taste with salt and pepper. Cover and refrigerate for 1 hour to blend the flavors.

Nutrients Per Serving	
Calories	150
Carbohydrate	22 g
Fiber	5 g
Protein	6 g
Fat	5 g
Iron	2 mg
Calcium	39 mg

Swiss Chard and Potato Salad

Getting bored of regular old potato salad? This one makes a great alternative.

Tips

If you prefer Swiss chard cooked very soft, add it with the potatoes and cook for a total of 20 minutes.

Spinach, endive or escarole can sub in for the Swiss chard, depending on what's in season. If using spinach, just add it for the last minute of cooking time so it wilts but doesn't overcook.

Leftovers of this salad taste great spread on top of toasted Brown Sandwich Bread (page 157).

2 cups	cubed potatoes (unpeeled)	500 mL
4 cups	chopped Swiss chard	1 L
2 tbsp	extra virgin olive oil	30 mL
	Salt and freshly ground black pepper	

1. Place potatoes in a large pot and cover with 8 cups (2 L) water. Bring to a boil over medium-high heat. Reduce heat and simmer for 15 minutes or until almost tender. Add Swiss chard and simmer for 5 to 8 minutes or until potatoes and chard are tender. Drain and transfer to a large bowl.

2. Drizzle chard and potatoes with oil, season with salt and pepper to taste and toss to coat.

Nutrients Per Serving	
Calories	230
Carbohydrate	38 g
Fiber	4 g
Protein	4 g
Fat	7 g
Iron	2 mg
Calcium	33 mg

Quinoa Salad

This simple, delicious salad packs a nutritional punch. Thanks to the quinoa (pronounced *keen-wah*), it even provides a complete protein, so it's a great choice for vegetarians. Whether it serves 2 people or 4 depends on how much you're willing to share!

Variation

If you're making this salad for non-vegetarians, you can substitute reduced-sodium GF chicken or turkey broth for the vegetable broth.

1 1/4 cups	reduced-sodium GF vegetable broth	300 mL
3/4 cup	quinoa, rinsed	175 mL
1/2 cup	thawed frozen peas	125 mL
1/4 cup	finely chopped orange bell pepper	60 mL
1/4 cup	finely chopped yellow bell pepper	60 mL
1 tbsp	finely chopped red onion	15 mL
2 tbsp	extra virgin olive oil	30 mL
1 tbsp	chopped fresh parsley	15 mL
1 tsp	dried thyme	5 mL
1 tsp	freshly squeezed lemon juice	5 mL
	Salt and freshly ground black pepper	

1. In a saucepan, bring broth to a boil over high heat. Add quinoa, reduce heat to low, cover and simmer for 20 minutes or until quinoa is tender and liquid is almost absorbed. Remove from heat and let stand, covered, for 5 minutes or until liquid is absorbed.

2. In a large bowl, combine quinoa, peas, orange pepper, yellow pepper and red onion.

3. In a small bowl, whisk together oil, parsley, thyme and lemon juice. Drizzle over salad and toss to coat. Season to taste with salt and pepper. Serve warm or cover and refrigerate for 1 hour, until chilled, and serve cold.

Nutrients Per Serving	
Calories	210
Carbohydrate	26 g
Fiber	4 g
Protein	6 g
Fat	9 g
Iron	2 mg
Calcium	32 mg

Quinoa Salad Niçoise

Makes 4 servings

This salad is great for summer picnics. Simply pack up all the elements individually and prepare the salad on a bed of romaine lettuce when you're ready to serve.

Tip

Choose canned "light" skipjack, yellowfin or tongol tuna. They contain less mercury than canned albacore tuna.

¾ cup	quinoa, rinsed	175 mL
2	eggs	2
4	romaine lettuce leaves	4
½ cup	chopped cooked GF ham	125 mL
¼ cup	chopped green olives	60 mL
¼ cup	chopped red onion	60 mL
½ cup	sliced roasted red bell pepper	125 mL
6	cherry tomatoes, sliced	6
1	can (6 oz/170 g) water-packed light tuna, drained	1
2 tbsp	extra virgin olive oil	30 mL
2 tbsp	white rice vinegar	30 mL
	Salt and freshly ground black pepper	

1. In a saucepan, bring 1¼ cups (300 mL) water to a boil over high heat. Add quinoa, reduce heat to low, cover and simmer for 20 minutes or until quinoa is tender and liquid is almost absorbed. Remove from heat and let stand, covered, for 5 minutes or until liquid is absorbed.

2. Meanwhile, place eggs in another saucepan and cover with water. Bring to a boil over high heat. Remove from heat, cover and let stand for 15 minutes. Peel off shells and cut eggs in half.

3. Arrange romaine lettuce in a large serving dish. Arrange quinoa evenly over lettuce, followed by eggs, ham, olives, red onion, roasted pepper, tomatoes and tuna. Drizzle with oil and vinegar. Season to taste with salt and pepper.

Nutrients Per Serving	
Calories	340
Carbohydrate	27 g
Fiber	4 g
Protein	24 g
Fat	15 g
Iron	4 mg
Calcium	65 mg

Spinach Salad with Chicken and Mandarin Oranges

Makes 4 servings

Theresa loves this salad so much she has a hard time sharing it. However, she's happy to share the recipe with you.

6 cups	packed baby spinach leaves (about 10 oz/300 g)	1.5 L
2 cups	chopped cooked chicken	500 mL
2 cups	bean sprouts (mung bean sprouts)	500 mL
½ cup	slivered almonds	125 mL
2	cans (each 10 oz/284 mL) mandarin oranges, drained	2
½ cup	light GF poppy seed dressing	125 mL

1. In a large bowl, combine spinach, chicken, bean sprouts, almonds and oranges. Add poppy seed dressing and toss to coat.

Nutrients Per Serving	
Calories	360
Carbohydrate	27 g
Fiber	5 g
Protein	28 g
Fat	16 g
Iron	3 mg
Calcium	104 mg

Egg Salad Roll-Ups

Theresa's sons, Eli and
Joseph, have always loved
her egg salad sandwiches.
The green olives make
them especially tasty.

Tip

If you already have
crêpes made, be sure to
microwave them on High
for 20 seconds before
assembling.

Variation

Instead of using the
crêpes, you can just use
the romaine leaves to
roll up the egg salad. It
also tastes great with
Brown Sandwich Bread
(page 157).

6	eggs	6
½ cup	sliced green olives	125 mL
½ cup	chopped celery	125 mL
¼ cup	chopped onion	60 mL
¼ cup	light GF mayonnaise	60 mL
1 tsp	prepared GF mustard	5 mL
4	Crêpes (see recipe, page 150)	4
4	romaine lettuce leaves	4

1. Place eggs in a medium saucepan and cover with water. Bring to a boil over high heat. Remove from heat, cover and let stand for 15 minutes. Peel off shells.

2. In a large bowl, mash eggs with a potato masher. Stir in olives, celery, onion, mayonnaise and mustard.

3. Line each crêpe with a romaine leaf. Spread one-quarter of the egg salad along the center of each leaf. Roll up and serve.

Nutrients Per Serving

Calories	280
Carbohydrate	18 g
Fiber	1 g
Protein	12 g
Fat	18 g
Iron	2 mg
Calcium	67 mg

Pizza and Pasta

Pizza Crust

Makes 8 rectangles
(1 rectangle per
serving)

Life quite simply must involve pizza, especially in Theresa's house. It is a weekly staple, as it is in many homes.

Tips

To make pizza, top with your favorite sauce and pizza toppings and broil for 5 to 10 minutes or until crust is crisp and toppings are bubbling, or follow the recipe on page 189.

Warm the milk in a glass measuring cup in the microwave on High for about 1 minute, or the traditional way, in a small saucepan over low heat.

This dough can also be made into a bread loaf. After making the dough, follow steps 3 and 4 of Brown Sandwich Bread (page 157).

Nutrients Per Serving	
Calories	210
Carbohydrate	29 g
Fiber	4 g
Protein	5 g
Fat	9 g
Iron	1 mg
Calcium	43 mg

- Stand mixer
- 15- by 10-inch (30 by 25 cm) rimmed baking sheet, lined with parchment paper

1 cup	white rice flour	250 mL
⅓ cup	psyllium husks	75 mL
¼ cup	sorghum flour	60 mL
¼ cup	brown rice flour	60 mL
¼ cup	tapioca starch or potato starch	60 mL
2 tbsp	granulated raw cane sugar	30 mL
1 tsp	salt	5 mL
¼ cup	grapeseed or olive oil	60 mL
2 tsp	instant yeast	10 mL
1 cup	lactose-free 1% milk, heated to 120°F to 130°F (50°C to 55°C)	250 mL
2	eggs, lightly beaten	2
	White rice flour	

1. In large bowl of stand mixer, combine white rice flour, psyllium, sorghum flour, brown rice flour, tapioca starch, sugar, salt and oil. Beat on low speed until oil is incorporated. Add yeast and beat for 1 minute.

2. With motor running on low, gradually pour in heated milk, beating until incorporated. Beat for 1 minute. Beat in eggs until incorporated. Beat for 5 minutes, stopping mixer and scraping down sides of bowl and beater halfway through.

3. Dust prepared baking sheet with white rice flour. Scoop or spoon batter onto baking sheet. With floured hands, shape dough into a circle. Lightly dust dough and rolling pin with rice flour. Roll out dough to evenly cover sheet. If necessary, use floured fingers to work the dough into the corners. Cover with a lint-free towel and let rise in a warm, draft-free place for 45 to 60 minutes or until doubled in bulk. Meanwhile, preheat oven to 350°F (180°C).

4. Bake for 15 to 20 minutes or until lightly browned and a tester inserted in the center comes out clean.

Pizza-Night Pizza

Friday nights were pizza and movie night at Theresa's house when her boys were growing up. It was almost always eaten in the living room, with a red checkered tablecloth placed on the floor in front of the television while a favorite movie played. Ah, the memories.

- Preheat broiler

1	baked Pizza Crust (see recipe, page 188)	1
½ cup	GF tomato sauce	125 mL
1 cup	shredded GF mozzarella-style rice cheese or part-skim mozzarella cheese	250 mL
¼ cup	grated Romano cheese	60 mL
6	slices prosciutto	6
20	green olives, sliced	20

1. Spread tomato sauce over crust on baking sheet, then sprinkle with mozzarella and Romano cheese. Arrange prosciutto and olives on top.

2. Broil for 5 to 10 minutes or until cheese is melted and bubbling.

Nutrients Per Serving	
Calories	290
Carbohydrate	32 g
Fiber	4 g
Protein	11 g
Fat	13 g
Iron	1 mg
Calcium	204 mg

After-School Pizza

This miniature pizza makes a nutritious after-school snack. These are also great at kids' birthday parties, because every child can create his or her own pizza from a selection of toppings you lay out for them. Adults like them too!

- Preheat broiler

1	plain GF rice cake	1
1 tbsp	GF ketchup	15 mL
1 to 2 tbsp	shredded mozzarella cheese or GF mozzarella-style rice cheese	15 to 30 mL
4	slices GF pepperoni	4
3	green olives, sliced	3
Pinch	dried Italian seasoning	Pinch

1. Spread ketchup evenly over rice cake and sprinkle with cheese to taste. Arrange pepperoni and olives on top. Sprinkle with Italian seasoning.

2. Broil for 40 to 60 seconds or until cheese is melted. Let cool.

Nutrients Per Serving	
Calories	140
Carbohydrate	13 g
Fiber	1 g
Protein	12 g
Fat	5 g
Iron	1 mg
Calcium	40 mg

Pasta with Shrimp and Peas

This quick and easy pasta recipe is ready in 30 minutes tops — perfect for those busy weeknights!

Tip

When Theresa saw Paul Newman showing Sally Field how to peel garlic in *Absence of Malice*, she decided to give it a try, and she's been peeling garlic that way ever since. Cut off the hard end of the clove, then lay a chef's knife on top of the clove so that the broad side is facing up. Making a fist, pound the knife with your hand. This loosens the peel so that it slips right off the clove. It also crushes the clove a bit, but that doesn't matter if you plan to mince it; in fact, it helps you on your way.

12 oz	GF penne or spiral pasta	375 g
3 tbsp	olive oil	45 mL
3 to 4	cloves garlic, minced	3 to 4
1 tsp	dried basil	5 mL
1 tsp	dried parsley	5 mL
Pinch	cayenne pepper	Pinch
8 oz	cooked peeled frozen shrimp	250 g
1 cup	frozen green peas	250 mL
¼ cup	grated Romano cheese	60 mL
	Salt and freshly ground black pepper	

1. In a large pot of boiling water, cook pasta according to package instructions until tender but firm (al dente). Drain, reserving 2 cups (500 mL) of the pasta cooking water. Return pasta to the pot.

2. In a skillet, heat oil over low heat. Sauté garlic to taste, basil, parsley and cayenne for 3 to 5 minutes or until garlic is softened and fragrant. Add shrimp and peas; sauté for about 5 minutes or until heated through.

3. Add shrimp mixture to pasta. Add enough of the reserved pasta cooking water to moisten to desired consistency, tossing gently to coat. Stir in Romano cheese and season to taste with salt and pepper.

Nutrients Per Serving	
Calories	360
Carbohydrate	46 g
Fiber	4 g
Protein	16 g
Fat	11 g
Iron	2 mg
Calcium	118 mg

Turkey Sausage and Spiral Pasta

Turkey sausage is a nice alternative to pork sausage. There are many choices out there; just make sure the sausages you choose are gluten-free.

Variation

Substitute GF pork or chicken sausage for the turkey sausage.

1 lb	turkey sausages (about 4), cut into chunks	500 g
5 tbsp	olive oil	75 mL
1	clove garlic, minced	1
1 cup	chopped broccoli	250 mL
1 cup	chopped celery	250 mL
½ cup	chopped red bell pepper	125 mL
½ cup	chopped onion	125 mL
1 tsp	dried basil	5 mL
1 tsp	dried parsley	5 mL
12 oz	GF brown rice spiral pasta	375 g
¼ cup	grated Romano cheese	60 mL

1. In a skillet, over medium-high heat, sauté sausage for 10 to 15 minutes or until browned on all sides and no longer pink inside. Using a slotted spoon, transfer to a plate lined with paper towels to drain. Pour off any fat from skillet.

2. Add oil to skillet and heat over medium-high heat. Sauté garlic, broccoli, celery, red pepper, onion, basil and parsley for 5 to 10 minutes or until tender-crisp.

3. Meanwhile, in a large pot of boiling water, cook pasta according to package instructions until tender but firm (al dente). Drain and transfer to a large bowl.

4. Add sausage and vegetable mixture to pasta and stir gently to combine. Serve sprinkled with Romano cheese.

Nutrients Per Serving	
Calories	380
Carbohydrate	45 g
Fiber	3 g
Protein	13 g
Fat	17 g
Iron	2 mg
Calcium	48 mg

Pasta Carbonara

This is Theresa's all-time favorite pasta. Enjoy it as she does, served with a tomato salad and a side of cooked peas, mushrooms and onions.

Tip

Use your favorite GF pasta for this recipe. Theresa particularly likes pasta made from a mix of quinoa and brown rice.

12 oz	GF spiral or penne pasta	375 g
8	slices bacon, chopped	8
3 tbsp	olive oil	45 mL
4 to 6	cloves garlic, minced	4 to 6
1 tbsp	chopped fresh parsley	15 mL
2	eggs, lightly beaten	2
1 cup	grated Romano cheese	250 mL

1. In a large pot of boiling water, cook pasta according to package instructions until tender but firm (al dente). Drain, reserving $1\frac{1}{2}$ cups (375 mL) of the pasta cooking water. Return pasta to the pot.

2. Meanwhile, in a skillet over medium heat, cook bacon, stirring, for about 5 minutes or until crisp. Using a slotted spoon, transfer to a plate lined with paper towels to drain. Pour off any fat from skillet.

3. Add oil to skillet and heat over medium heat. Sauté garlic to taste and parsley for 2 to 3 minutes or until garlic is golden. Add to pasta.

4. In a small bowl, whisk together eggs and cheese. Pour over pasta. Place pot over low heat and cook, stirring constantly, for 3 to 5 minutes or until eggs thicken. Add enough of the reserved pasta cooking water to moisten to desired consistency, tossing gently to coat. Stir in bacon.

Nutrients Per Serving

Calories	450
Carbohydrate	52 g
Fiber	1 g
Protein	15 g
Fat	18 g
Iron	4 mg
Calcium	289 mg

Spaghetti and Meatballs

Makes 6 to 8 servings

This sauce is a little time-consuming, but oh so worth it. Make it on the weekend, when you have time to putter and enjoy a great meal at the end of the day. Serve with cooked rapini and red peppers, with a salad on the side. Any accolades for this recipe go to Theresa's mom.

Tip

If you're out of GF dry bread crumbs, use a blender or food processor to grind GF crackers or GF rice cakes to fine crumbs.

Variation

Substitute 1 lb (500 g) whole GF turkey sausages for the meatballs. Cook whole sausages in the sauce and cut into pieces before serving. Or use a combination of both.

Nutrients Per Serving	
Calories	430
Carbohydrate	61 g
Fiber	6 g
Protein	21 g
Fat	10 g
Iron	4 mg
Calcium	185 mg

1 lb	extra-lean ground beef	500 g
½ cup	chopped onion	125 mL
½ cup	GF dry bread crumbs	125 mL
½ cup	grated Romano cheese	125 mL
2 tbsp	chopped fresh parsley	30 mL
1 tbsp	grated lemon zest	15 mL
1 tsp	dried Italian seasoning	5 mL
1 tsp	dried basil	5 mL
2 tsp	olive oil	10 mL
1	can (28 oz/796 mL) crushed tomatoes	1
1	jar (23 oz/650 mL) GF spinach-and-cheese-flavored tomato pasta sauce	1
1 lb	GF spaghetti	500 g

1. In a large bowl, using your hands, combine beef, onion, bread crumbs, cheese, parsley, lemon zest, Italian seasoning and basil. Scoop up 2 tbsp (30 mL) beef mixture and form into a ball. Repeat until all the beef mixture is formed into meatballs.

2. In a large saucepan, heat oil over medium-high heat. Cook meatballs, turning often, until browned on all sides. Stir in tomatoes, pasta sauce and 3 cups (750 mL) water; bring to a boil. Cover, leaving lid ajar, reduce heat to low and simmer for 2½ hours to blend the flavors.

3. In a large pot of boiling water, cook spaghetti according to package instructions until tender but firm (al dente). Drain and transfer to a serving platter.

4. Ladle meatballs and sauce over spaghetti.

Eggplant and Zucchini Lasagna

Theresa has tried many times to be a vegetarian, but the men in her household prefer meat lasagna. So this is a lasagna solely for her. She will share it, but only if you ask nicely.

Tip

If you need to avoid dairy foods, you can replace the ricotta cheese and mozzarella cheese with 3 cups (750 mL) shredded GF mozzarella-style rice cheese.

- Preheat oven to 350°F (180°C)
- 13- by 9-inch (33 by 23 cm) glass baking dish

9	GF lasagna noodles	9
1	jar (23 oz/650 mL) GF tomato pasta sauce, preferably with spinach	1
1½ cups	shredded part-skim mozzarella cheese	375 mL
1	Japanese eggplant, thinly sliced	1
1½ cups	light ricotta cheese	375 mL
1	zucchini, thinly sliced	1
¼ cup	grated Romano cheese	60 mL
	Salt and freshly ground black pepper	

1. In a large pot of boiling water, cook lasagna according to package instructions until tender but firm (al dente). Drain.

2. Spread a thin layer of pasta sauce in baking dish. Top with 3 lasagna noodles, making sure they don't overlap. Cover with one-quarter of the sauce. Sprinkle with one-third of the mozzarella. Arrange eggplant on top. Cover with one-third of the remaining sauce, then half the ricotta. Add 3 more noodles and top with layers of tomato sauce and half the remaining mozzarella. Arrange zucchini on top. Cover with the remaining sauce, then the remaining ricotta. Top with the remaining noodles.

3. Pour ½ cup (125 mL) water into the pasta sauce jar and swish to catch any remaining sauce; pour over lasagna. Sprinkle with the remaining mozzarella and Romano cheese.

4. Cover with foil and bake in preheated oven for 45 to 50 minutes or until sauce is bubbling and cheese is melted. Remove foil and bake for 15 minutes. Broil for 5 minutes or until top is browned. Let stand for 10 minutes before serving. Season to taste with salt and pepper.

Nutrients Per Serving

Calories	370
Carbohydrate	45 g
Fiber	7 g
Protein	19 g
Fat	15 g
Iron	2 mg
Calcium	430 mg

Lasagna with Meat Sauce

Theresa's son Joseph loves meat in his tomato sauce, so she makes this meat sauce especially for him.

Tip

If any of the noodles break, use them for the bottom of the lasagna and save the perfect ones for the top layer — no one will notice.

Variation

You can use ground turkey instead of beef.

- Preheat oven to 350°F (180°C)
- 13- by 9-inch (33 by 23 cm) glass baking dish, greased

12	brown rice lasagna noodles	12
2 tsp	olive oil	10 mL
1 lb	extra-lean ground beef	500 g
1 cup	chopped onion	250 mL
1	clove garlic, minced	1
1	jar (23 oz/650 mL) GF tomato pasta sauce, preferably with spinach	1
1½ cups	shredded part-skim mozzarella cheese	375 mL
1¼ cups	grated Romano or Parmesan cheese	300 mL

1. In a large pot of boiling water, cook lasagna according to package instructions until tender but firm (al dente). Drain.

2. In a large saucepan, heat oil over medium-high heat. Cook beef, onion and garlic, breaking beef up with the back of a spoon, for about 8 minutes or until beef is no longer pink. Stir in pasta sauce and cook, stirring and scraping up any brown bits stuck to pan, for about 3 minutes or until sauce is bubbling. Remove from heat.

3. Spread a thin layer of pasta sauce in prepared baking dish. Top with 3 lasagna noodles, making sure they don't overlap. Cover with one-quarter of the sauce. Sprinkle with one-quarter each of the mozzarella and Romano. Repeat layers three more times, ending with cheeses.

4. Cover with foil and bake in preheated oven for 45 to 50 minutes or until sauce is bubbling and cheese is melted. Remove foil and bake for 15 minutes or until top is lightly browned. Let stand for 10 minutes before serving.

Nutrients Per Serving

Calories	360
Carbohydrate	32 g
Fiber	3 g
Protein	23 g
Fat	14 g
Iron	2 mg
Calcium	386 mg

Vegetarian Mains and Seafood

Mushroom Casserole

Theresa's mother-in-law often served a dish similar to this one. Theresa has used gluten-free ingredients, but the great taste remains the same.

Tip

Vegan hard margarine, such as Earth Balance vegan buttery flavor sticks, has almost half as much saturated fat as regular butter and no cholesterol. Where butter is called for in a recipe, vegan hard margarine can be a heart-healthy, delicious alternative.

Variations

If you're feeding this dish to non-vegetarians, you can nestle 4 boneless skinless chicken thighs into the rice in the baking dish.

Substitute chopped broccoli for the peas.

- Preheat oven to 350°F (180°C)
- 10- by 8-inch (25 by 20 cm) casserole dish

1 tbsp	grapeseed oil	15 mL
1 tbsp	vegan hard margarine or butter	15 mL
8 oz	mushrooms, sliced	250 g
1/2 cup	frozen peas	125 mL
1/3 cup	chopped celery	75 mL
1 tsp	white rice flour	5 mL
1 1/3 cups	fortified GF non-dairy milk or lactose-free 1% milk	325 mL
1/3 cup	long-grain brown rice	75 mL
1/3 cup	quinoa, rinsed	75 mL
1 tbsp	GF soy sauce	15 mL

1. In a skillet, heat oil and margarine over medium heat. Sauté mushrooms, peas and celery for 5 to 10 minutes or until mushrooms are golden brown and slightly crispy. Sprinkle with flour and stir until blended. Gradually stir in milk.

2. Pour mushroom mixture into baking dish and stir in rice, quinoa and soy sauce.

3. Cover and bake in preheated oven for 45 to 50 minutes or until rice and quinoa are tender and most of the liquid is absorbed.

Nutrients Per Serving	
Calories	320
Carbohydrate	40 g
Fiber	4 g
Protein	11 g
Fat	12 g
Iron	3 mg
Calcium	190 mg

Zucchini Patties

Theresa's sons used to call these "cheese patties" because they preferred not to think about the fact that there's zucchini in them. The patties are fantastic as either a main dish or a side dish, and either hot or cold.

- Spray bottle of grapeseed oil

4	eggs, beaten	4
4	cloves garlic, minced	4
2 cups	shredded zucchini	500 mL
½ cup	shredded mozzarella cheese or mozzarella-style rice cheese	125 mL
½ cup	shredded reduced-fat Cheddar cheese or Cheddar-style rice cheese	125 mL
½ cup	sorghum flour or white rice flour	125 mL
	Salt and freshly ground black pepper	

1. In a large bowl, combine eggs, garlic, zucchini, mozzarella, Cheddar and flour.

2. Spray a large skillet with oil and heat over medium-high heat. For each patty, pour in ¼ cup (60 mL) batter. Cook for 1 to 2 minutes or until edges are firm. Flip over and cook for 1 to 2 minutes or until golden and hot in the center. Transfer to a plate and keep warm. Repeat with the remaining batter, spraying skillet with oil and adjusting heat between batches as needed.

Nutrients Per Serving

Calories	200
Carbohydrate	20 g
Fiber	2 g
Protein	14 g
Fat	8 g
Iron	2 mg
Calcium	180 mg

Quinoa Cashew Oven Pilaf

Theresa's friend Christine served this delicious dish one summer day at a picnic and was kind enough to share her recipe. Theresa adapted it for you. If you prefer to serve it as a side dish rather than a main course, it will serve 8.

Tip

Choose your favorite GF non-dairy milk, such as soy, rice, almond or potato-based milk, for this recipe.

- Preheat oven to 350°F (180°C)
- 10- by 8-inch (25 by 20 cm) casserole dish, lightly greased

1	clove garlic, minced	1
¾ cup	chopped raw cashews	175 mL
½ cup	chopped onion	125 mL
½ cup	chopped celery	125 mL
½ cup	chopped red bell pepper	125 mL
½ cup	quinoa, rinsed	125 mL
1½ cups	fortified GF non-dairy milk	375 mL
1 tbsp	chopped fresh parsley	15 mL
1 tsp	dried basil	5 mL
¼ tsp	dried sage	1 mL
	Salt and freshly ground black pepper	

1. In a large bowl, combine garlic, cashews, onion, celery, red pepper and quinoa. Stir in milk, parsley, basil and sage. Season to taste with salt and pepper. Pour into prepared baking dish.

2. Bake in preheated oven for about 45 minutes or until golden and liquid is absorbed. Spoon onto serving plates.

Nutrients Per Serving	
Calories	290
Carbohydrate	30 g
Fiber	3 g
Protein	10 g
Fat	15 g
Iron	4 mg
Calcium	174 mg

Polenta with Tomato Sauce

Makes 2 servings

This is Theresa's version of her mom's polenta. In her parents' era, this meal was served on a large board in the middle of the dinner table. Everyone had a fork and dug in. Now that's Theresa's kind of eating.

Tip

Look for a tomato pasta sauce with a reduced sodium content, ideally 330 to 390 mg per ½-cup (125 mL) serving.

1 tbsp	grapeseed oil	15 mL
6	¼-inch (0.5 cm) thick slices prepared polenta	6
1 cup	GF tomato pasta sauce	250 mL
½ cup	grated Romano cheese	125 mL

1. In a large skillet, heat oil over medium-high heat. Cook polenta slices for about 1 minute per side or until golden. Add tomato sauce and cook for 1 minute. Reduce heat and simmer for 5 minutes. Serve sprinkled with cheese.

Nutrients Per Serving	
Calories	290
Carbohydrate	30 g
Fiber	3 g
Protein	10 g
Fat	14 g
Iron	4 mg
Calcium	174 mg

Teff Polenta

Makes 4 servings

This recipe is from *Going Wild in the Kitchen* by Leslie Cerier (Square One Publishers, 2005). Used with permission.

Tip

At the end of step 1, there may be some extra liquid from the tomatoes, but as long as the teff is not crunchy, the polenta is done.

- 10-inch (25 cm) skillet
- 9-inch (23 cm) pie plate

2 tbsp	extra virgin olive oil	30 mL
8	cloves garlic, thickly sliced	8
1 cup	coarsely chopped onion	250 mL
1 cup	chopped green bell pepper	250 mL
2/3 cup	teff grain	150 mL
2 cups	boiling water	500 mL
1/2 tsp	sea salt	2 mL
2 cups	chopped plum (Roma) tomatoes	500 mL
1 cup	chopped fresh basil	250 mL

1. In skillet, heat oil over medium heat. Sauté garlic and onion for 5 minutes or until tender. Add green pepper and sauté for 2 minutes or until bright green. Stir in teff flour. Gradually stir in boiling water and salt; simmer, stirring, for 2 minutes. Stir in tomatoes and basil; reduce heat to low, cover and simmer, stirring occasionally, for 10 to 15 minutes or until water is absorbed.

2. Transfer polenta to pie plate and let cool for 30 minutes before slicing and serving.

Nutrients Per Serving	
Calories	220
Carbohydrate	32 g
Fiber	6 g
Protein	6 g
Fat	8 g
Iron	3 mg
Calcium	102 mg

Tofu Stir-Fry

Makes 4 servings

Many people think they don't like tofu, but this dish will change their minds! There's no need to tell them before they eat it — just let them gobble it down, then surprise them with the reveal.

Tip

To save time, you can use 6 cups (1.5 L) frozen chopped vegetables, thawed.

• Blender

6 oz	firm tofu	175 g
2 tbsp	natural peanut butter	30 mL
2 tbsp	GF soy sauce	30 mL
2 tbsp	grapeseed oil	30 mL
1 cup	green beans, trimmed	250 mL
1 cup	snow peas, trimmed	250 mL
1 cup	chopped broccoli	250 mL
1 cup	chopped celery	250 mL
1/2 cup	chopped red bell pepper	125 mL
1/2 cup	chopped yellow bell pepper	125 mL
1/2 cup	sliced or chopped zucchini	125 mL
1/4 cup	chopped red onion	60 mL
1	clove garlic, minced	1
1/2 cup	raw cashews	125 mL

1. In blender, combine tofu, peanut butter, soy sauce and 1/4 cup (60 mL) water; blend until smooth. Set aside.

2. In a wok or a large skillet, heat oil over medium-high heat. Stir-fry beans, snow peas, broccoli, celery, red pepper, yellow pepper, zucchini, red onion and garlic for 5 minutes. Stir in tofu mixture and stir-fry for 5 to 10 minutes or until vegetables are tender-crisp (or cook to desired doneness). Serve sprinkled with cashews.

Nutrients Per Serving	
Calories	340
Carbohydrate	24 g
Fiber	7 g
Protein	16 g
Fat	23 g
Iron	4 mg
Calcium	349 mg

Battered Fish

Theresa and her family love to fish. They catch perch all summer long and never tire of eating it with this batter, which is light and fluffy and tastes a bit like potato chips. It can be used for any kind of fish, for shrimp or even for onion rings.

Tip

Extra fried fish fillets can be cooled on a wire rack, wrapped in parchment paper and frozen in an airtight container or freezer bag for up to 2 months. Place frozen fish on a baking sheet lined with parchment paper or foil and reheat in a 400°F (200°C) oven for 20 minutes, flipping over halfway through, until fish is heated through and batter is crispy.

1/2 cup	white rice flour	125 mL
1/2 cup	sorghum flour or additional white rice flour	125 mL
1 tsp	salt	5 mL
1/4 tsp	freshly ground black pepper	1 mL
2	eggs, separated	2
3/4 cup	GF beer or water	175 mL
1 tbsp	butter or vegan hard margarine, melted	15 mL
1/4 cup	grapeseed oil (approx.)	60 mL
8	pieces skinless white fish fillets (each about 3 1/2 oz/100 g)	8

1. In a large bowl, combine rice flour, sorghum flour, salt and pepper.

2. In a small bowl, whisk together egg yolks, beer and butter. Stir in flour mixture.

3. In another bowl, using an electric mixer, beat egg whites until firm peaks form. Fold into flour mixture.

4. In a large skillet, heat oil over medium-high heat. Dip fish fillets in batter, one at a time, shaking off and discarding excess batter. In batches as necessary to avoid crowding pan, fry fish for 4 to 5 minutes per side or until fish flakes easily when tested with a fork, adding more oil and adjusting heat between batches as necessary.

Nutrients Per Serving	
Calories	300
Carbohydrate	14 g
Fiber	1 g
Protein	25 g
Fat	15 g
Iron	1 mg
Calcium	36 mg

Fish for the Sole

You'll forgive the pun, we hope, but this cracker-crusted fish really is comfort food for the soul — and it does your body good, too!

Tip

To crush the crackers, place them in a sealable plastic bag. Seal and use a rolling pin to crush them to the consistency of dry bread crumbs. Alternatively, you can crush them in a blender.

- Preheat oven to 350°F (180°C)
- 13- by 9-inch (33 by 23 cm) glass baking dish, greased

2	cloves garlic, minced	2
$1/4$ cup	GF cracker crumbs	60 mL
2 tbsp	chopped fresh parsley	30 mL
2 tbsp	olive oil (approx.)	30 mL
	Juice of $1/2$ lemon	
3	pieces skinless sole fillet (each about $3^1/_2$ oz/100 g)	3

1. In a small bowl, combine garlic, cracker crumbs, parsley, oil and lemon juice; stir until a paste forms, adding more oil if mixture is too dry.

2. Arrange sole in prepared baking dish. Spread paste over fish.

3. Cover dish with foil and bake in preheated oven for 20 to 30 minutes or until fish flakes easily when tested with a fork. Uncover and bake for 5 minutes or until crust is crispy.

Nutrients Per Serving	
Calories	220
Carbohydrate	8 g
Fiber	1 g
Protein	23 g
Fat	10 g
Iron	1 mg
Calcium	41 mg

Baked Salmon Patties

These patties are so darn good, it's difficult to eat just one — so have two!

Tips

If you prefer, you can remove the bones from the salmon, but they contribute a significant amount of calcium. If you remove them, each serving will provide just 24 mg calcium.

In addition to making cleanup easier, parchment paper is biodegradable.

- Preheat oven to 350°F (180°C)
- Rimmed baking sheet, lined with parchment paper

2	cans (each 6 oz/170 g) salmon, drained	2
1	egg, beaten	1
1 cup	shredded reduced-fat Cheddar cheese	250 mL
1 cup	finely chopped celery	250 mL
1/4 cup	finely chopped onion	60 mL
2 tsp	chopped fresh parsley	10 mL
	Juice of 1/2 lemon	

1. In a large bowl, mash salmon with a fork, crushing the bones. Stir in egg, cheese, celery, onion, parsley and lemon juice until well combined. Using your hands, form mixture into eight 1/2-inch (1 cm) thick patties.

2. Place on prepared baking sheet and bake in preheated oven for 20 minutes. Flip patties over and bake for 10 minutes or until golden brown and hot in the center.

Nutrients Per Serving	
Calories	190
Carbohydrate	3 g
Fiber	1 g
Protein	28 g
Fat	7 g
Iron	1 mg
Calcium	372 mg

Trout with Walnuts

Theresa's husband loves to fish for trout, and this is one of his favorite ways to eat it.

Tip

Vegan hard margarine, such as Earth Balance vegan buttery flavor sticks, has almost half as much saturated fat as regular butter and no cholesterol. Where butter is called for in a recipe, vegan hard margarine can be a heart-healthy, delicious alternative.

1 tbsp	grapeseed oil	15 mL
1 tbsp	vegan hard margarine or butter	15 mL
1	skin-on trout fillet (about 8 oz/250 g), cut in half	1
	Juice of ½ lemon	
	Salt and freshly ground black pepper	
¼ cup	chopped walnuts	60 mL
	Lemon slices	

1. In a large skillet, heat oil and margarine over medium-high heat. Add fish, skin side up, and cook for 5 minutes per side or until fish flakes easily when tested with a fork.

2. Transfer fish to a serving platter. Drizzle with lemon juice and season to taste with salt and pepper. Sprinkle with walnuts and garnish with lemon slices.

Nutrients Per Serving	
Calories	300
Carbohydrate	3 g
Fiber	1 g
Protein	21 g
Fat	23 g
Iron	1 mg
Calcium	35 mg

Tuna Casserole

Tuna casseroles are among the easiest meals to prepare. This tasty version has added protein and flavor thanks to the quinoa. Enjoy it with a salad on the side.

Tip

Vegan hard margarine, such as Earth Balance vegan buttery flavor sticks, has almost half as much saturated fat as regular butter and no cholesterol. Where butter is called for in a recipe, vegan hard margarine can be a heart-healthy, delicious alternative.

Variation

Add ½ cup (125 mL) frozen peas with the rice.

- Preheat oven to 350°F (180°C)
- 10- by 8-inch (25 by 20 cm) casserole dish with lid, lightly greased

1 tsp	grapeseed oil	5 mL
1 cup	chopped onion	250 mL
1 cup	chopped celery	250 mL
1 tbsp	chopped fresh parsley	15 mL
1 tsp	vegan hard margarine or butter	5 mL
1	can (6 oz/170 g) water-packed flaked tuna, drained	1
½ cup	long-grain brown rice	125 mL
½ cup	quinoa, rinsed	125 mL
2 cups	fortified GF non-dairy milk or lactose-free 1% milk	500 mL

1. In a skillet, heat oil over medium-high heat. Sauté onion, celery and parsley for 3 to 5 minutes or until onion is starting to brown. Stir in margarine. Remove from heat.

2. In prepared baking dish, combine tuna, rice, quinoa and milk. Stir in onion mixture.

3. Cover and bake in preheated oven for 45 minutes or until rice and quinoa are tender and liquid is absorbed. Uncover and bake for 5 minutes or until top is browned.

Nutrients Per Serving

Calories	300
Carbohydrate	39 g
Fiber	3 g
Protein	19 g
Fat	7 g
Iron	3 mg
Calcium	210 mg

Tuna Patties

Sometimes simple really is best — this recipe is proof!

2	cans (6 oz/170 g) water-packed flaked tuna, drained	2
2	eggs, beaten	2
¼ cup	potato starch	60 mL
½ cup	frozen peas, cooked, drained and mashed	125 mL
½ cup	finely chopped celery	125 mL
¼ cup	finely chopped red onion	60 mL
¼ cup	chopped roasted red bell peppers	60 mL
1 tbsp	grapeseed oil (approx.)	15 mL

1. In a large bowl, combine tuna, eggs, potato starch, peas, celery, red onion and roasted peppers. Using your hands, form mixture into eight ½-inch (1 cm) thick patties and place on a plate.

2. In a large skillet, heat oil over medium-high heat. Working in batches to avoid crowding, use a pancake flipper to carefully place patties in pan. Cook patties for 3 to 4 minutes per side or until browned and hot in the center, adding oil and adjusting heat as necessary between batches.

Nutrients Per Serving

Calories	230
Carbohydrate	16 g
Fiber	2 g
Protein	26 g
Fat	7 g
Iron	2 mg
Calcium	37 mg

Crustless Rapini and Clam Quiche

Theresa's sister, Linda, gave
her the idea of combining
rapini with clams, and the
result is this quiche, a great
choice for brunch or a
light supper.

Tip

Trim off the tough stems
from the rapini before
chopping and measuring.

- Preheat oven to 375°F (190°C)
- 9-inch (23 cm) glass pie plate, lightly greased

5 cups	chopped trimmed rapini	1.25 L
1 tbsp	grapeseed oil	15 mL
1 tsp	butter	5 mL
1	clove garlic, minced	1
½ cup	chopped red onion	125 mL
4	eggs	4
1½ cups	light ricotta cheese	375 mL
½ cup	grated Romano cheese	125 mL
1	can (5 oz/142 g) baby clams, drained	1

1. In a large pot of boiling salted water, cook rapini for
   10 to 15 minutes or until tender. Drain and set aside.

2. In a large skillet, heat oil and butter over medium-
   high heat. Sauté garlic and red onion for 3 to
   5 minutes or until soft and golden. Let cool slightly.

3. In a large bowl, whisk eggs until blended. Whisk
   in ricotta and Romano cheese. Stir in rapini, onion
   mixture and clams. Spread evenly in prepared
   pie plate.

4. Bake in preheated oven for 45 minutes or until set,
   puffed and golden. Let stand for 10 minutes before
   cutting.

Nutrients Per Serving	
Calories	210
Carbohydrate	7 g
Fiber	1 g
Protein	16 g
Fat	13 g
Iron	8 mg
Calcium	284 mg

Meat and Poultry

Oven-Baked Beef Stew

Makes 4 servings

This stew is full of flavor —
including the woodsy taste
of thyme, one of Theresa's
favorite herbs. Serve it up
with mashed potatoes or
over cooked rice, GF pasta
or quinoa.

- Preheat oven to 350°F (180°C)
- 8-inch (20 cm) glass baking dish

1 tbsp	grapeseed oil	15 mL
1 lb	lean stewing beef, cut into bite-size pieces	500 g
3	cloves garlic, minced	3
½ cup	chopped onion	125 mL
2 tsp	dried parsley	10 mL
1 tsp	dried thyme	5 mL
1 tbsp	white rice flour	15 mL
1¼ cups	reduced-sodium GF vegetable broth	300 mL
2 tsp	butter	10 mL
	Salt and freshly ground black pepper	

1. In a large skillet, heat oil over medium-high heat. Cook beef for 5 minutes or until browned on all sides. Using a slotted spoon, transfer to baking dish.

2. Reduce heat to medium. Add garlic, onion, parsley and thyme to skillet; sauté for 3 to 4 minutes or until onion is softened. Sprinkle with flour and cook, stirring, for 1 minute. Gradually stir in broth and bring to a boil, scraping up any brown bits from pan. Stir in butter until melted. Pour over beef.

3. Cover and bake in preheated oven for 1 hour or until meat is fork-tender. Season to taste with salt and pepper.

Nutrients Per Serving	
Calories	230
Carbohydrate	6 g
Fiber	2 g
Protein	26 g
Fat	11 g
Iron	3 mg
Calcium	55 mg

Fatina (Italian-Style Schnitzel)

Find a butcher who is willing to slice your eye of the round roast into thin slices. If you're able, buy the whole round and have him package it according to how many you want in each package. Then freeze until you decide to make these very tempting schnitzels. Let the beef thaw in the refrigerator overnight.

Tips

If the crackers you use have salt, do not add salt to the egg mixture.

For added fiber and nutrients, try using GF multigrain crackers, such as Mary's Gone Crackers, original or black pepper flavor.

If you find that the egg mixture is running low before you've dipped all the beef, add 1 tbsp (15 mL) water and stir.

Nutrients Per Serving	
Calories	380
Carbohydrate	17 g
Fiber	3 g
Protein	31 g
Fat	20 g
Iron	3 mg
Calcium	153 mg

1	egg	1
	Salt and freshly ground black pepper	
1 cup	GF cracker crumbs (see tip, page 205) or bread crumbs	250 mL
¼ cup	grated Romano cheese	60 mL
	Grated zest of 1 lemon	
1 lb	beef eye of round, cut into ⅛-inch (3 mm) slices	500 g
¼ cup	grapeseed oil (approx.)	60 mL
1	lemon, sliced	1

1. In a bowl, lightly beat egg. Season with salt and pepper.

2. In a shallow dish, combine cracker crumbs, cheese and lemon zest.

3. Working with one piece at a time, dip beef in egg mixture, then press into crumb mixture, coating evenly and shaking off excess. Discard any excess egg mixture and crumb mixture.

4. In a large skillet, heat 1 tbsp (15 mL) oil over medium-high heat. Working in batches of two or three pieces each, cook beef for 2 to 3 minutes per side or until coating is golden brown and beef is cooked to desired doneness. Transfer to a plate lined with paper towels. Add oil and adjust heat as necessary between batches.

5. Serve on a large platter, surrounded by lemon slices.

Skillet Shepherd's Pie

Makes 4 servings

Theresa loves to cook, but it's certainly a bonus when there's hardly any cleanup. Here's a recipe that fits the bill.

Tips

Whenever you can, try to use beef from locally raised, grass-fed cattle.

Choose your favorite GF non-dairy milk, such as soy, rice or potato-based milk or, if you tolerate lactose, use regular 1% milk.

Theresa's family likes the frozen vegetable combination of small-cut carrots, corn, beans and peas.

You can leave the skins on the potatoes if you prefer. It adds more fiber to the dish and makes it look hearty and comforting.

- Large ovenproof skillet

1 lb	potatoes, peeled and chopped	500 g
¼ cup	fortified GF non-dairy milk or lactose-free 1% milk	60 mL
2 tbsp	vegan hard margarine or butter	30 mL
1 cup	shredded reduced-fat Cheddar cheese or Cheddar-style rice cheese	250 mL
1 lb	extra-lean ground beef	500 g
½ cup	chopped onion	125 mL
1	clove garlic, minced	1
1 tbsp	chopped fresh parsley	15 mL
2 tsp	dried basil	10 mL
1 cup	frozen mixed vegetables	250 mL

1. Place potatoes in a large pot and add enough water to cover. Bring to a boil over high heat. Reduce heat to medium-low and boil for 15 to 20 minutes or until potatoes are tender.

2. Drain potatoes and return to pot. Add milk and margarine; using a potato masher, mash potatoes until smooth. Stir in cheese and set aside.

3. In ovenproof skillet, cook beef over medium-high heat, breaking it up with the back of a spoon, for 7 minutes or until no longer pink. Add onion, garlic, parsley and basil; cook, stirring, for 3 to 4 minutes or until tender. Add mixed vegetables and cook, stirring, for 5 minutes. Meanwhile, preheat broiler.

4. Spread mashed potatoes on top of beef mixture. Broil for 5 to 10 minutes or until potatoes are golden.

Nutrients Per Serving	
Calories	370
Carbohydrate	31 g
Fiber	4 g
Protein	32 g
Fat	13 g
Iron	3 mg
Calcium	177 mg

Salsa Burgers

Summer wouldn't be summer without salsa burgers. Serve them with GF hamburger buns and lay out assorted condiments and a platter of sliced tomatoes, sliced onions and lettuce leaves so everyone can garnish as desired.

- Preheat oven to 350°F (180°C)
- Rimmed baking sheet, lined with parchment paper

1 lb	extra-lean ground beef	500 g
½ cup	salsa	125 mL
½ cup	shredded part-skim mozzarella cheese	125 mL

1. In a large bowl, using your hands, combine beef, salsa and cheese until well blended. Form into four ½-inch (1 cm) thick patties and place on prepared baking sheet.

2. Bake in preheated oven for 15 to 20 minutes, turning halfway through, until a meat thermometer inserted in the middle of a burger registers 160°F (71°C). Use a slotted lifter to remove patties from baking sheet; discard excess liquid.

Nutrients Per Serving

Calories	180
Carbohydrate	3 g
Fiber	0 g
Protein	26 g
Fat	7 g
Iron	2 mg
Calcium	103 mg

Meatloaf

This recipe is based on
Theresa's grandmother's
meatloaf, often served at
her bed-and-breakfast in
Italy. The secret ingredient,
of course, is love.

Tips

For added fiber and
nutrients, try using GF
multigrain crackers, such
as Mary's Gone Crackers.
For extra-flavor, use herbed
GF crackers.

To crush the crackers,
place them in a sealable
plastic bag. Seal and use
a rolling pin to crush them
to the consistency of dry
bread crumbs. Alternatively,
you can crush them in a
blender.

Nutrients Per Serving	
Calories	260
Carbohydrate	3 g
Fiber	1 g
Protein	24 g
Fat	17 g
Iron	2 mg
Calcium	78 mg

- Preheat oven to 350°F (180°C)
- 9-inch (23 cm) round baking dish with lid, lightly greased.

1 lb	extra-lean ground beef	500 g
1 lb	lean ground veal	500 g
1 lb	lean ground pork	500 g
$\frac{1}{2}$ cup	grated Romano cheese	125 mL
$\frac{1}{4}$ cup	GF cracker crumbs	60 mL
3 tbsp	chopped fresh parsley	45 mL
2	eggs, lightly beaten	2
$\frac{2}{3}$ cup	tomato sauce, divided	150 mL
2 tbsp	olive oil	30 mL
	Grated zest of 1 lemon	

1. In a very large bowl, using your hands, combine beef, veal, pork, cheese, crackers, parsley, eggs, $\frac{1}{2}$ cup (125 mL) of the tomato sauce, oil and lemon zest. Knead until mixture is smooth and well combined. Form into a 9- by 5-inch (23 by 12.5 cm) loaf. Place in prepared baking dish and drizzle the remaining tomato sauce across the top.

2. Cover and bake in preheated oven for $1\frac{1}{2}$ hours or until a meat thermometer inserted in the center of the meatloaf registers 160°F (71°C). Let stand for 10 minutes before cutting into slices.

Veal Stew

Theresa's sons always make sure they're home for dinner when she's serving this stew. It's their all-time favorite meal, especially when served over Nokedli (page 237). It's also delicious over cooked rice or GF pasta.

Tip

This stew is quite saucy — perfect for soaking into the nokedli or rice or GF pasta.

2 tsp	grapeseed oil	10 mL
1 lb	stewing veal, cut into bite-size pieces	500 g
1	onion, chopped	1
1	red bell pepper, chopped	1
1	clove garlic, minced	1
2 tsp	paprika	10 mL
¼ tsp	cayenne pepper, or to taste	1 mL
4 cups	reduced-sodium GF chicken broth	1 L
	Salt and freshly ground black pepper	

1. In a large saucepan, heat oil over medium-high heat. Cook veal for 5 minutes or until browned on all sides. Using a slotted spoon, transfer to a plate.

2. Reduce heat to medium. Add onion, red pepper, garlic, paprika and cayenne to pan; sauté for 3 to 4 minutes or until vegetables are softened. Stir in broth and bring to a boil, scraping up any brown bits from pan.

3. Return veal and any accumulated juices to pan. Reduce heat to low, cover and simmer, stirring occasionally, for 45 to 60 minutes or until veal is fork-tender. Season to taste with salt and black pepper.

Nutrients Per Serving	
Calories	190
Carbohydrate	8 g
Fiber	2 g
Protein	26 g
Fat	6 g
Iron	2 mg
Calcium	32 mg

Chicken Cacciatore

Traditionally, chicken cacciatore is made with mushrooms. But Theresa's family prefers it without. If you wish, add 1 cup (250 mL) sliced mushrooms when sautéing the vegetables. Serve with Savory Tea Biscuits (page 161) or Popovers (page 159) or over cooked rice or GF spiral pasta.

2 tsp	grapeseed oil	10 mL
1½ lbs	boneless skinless chicken thighs	750 g
½ cup	chopped onion	125 mL
½ cup	chopped red bell pepper	125 mL
½ cup	chopped yellow bell pepper	125 mL
1 tsp	dried thyme	5 mL
1 tsp	dried basil	5 mL
1 tsp	dried marjoram	5 mL
2 cups	reduced-sodium GF chicken or vegetable broth	500 mL
½ cup	tomato sauce	125 mL
	Salt and freshly ground black pepper	

1. In a large saucepan, heat oil over medium-high heat. Cook chicken for 5 minutes per side or until browned on both sides.

2. Reduce heat to medium. Add onion, red pepper, yellow pepper, thyme, basil and marjoram; sauté for 3 to 4 minutes or until softened.

3. Stir in broth and tomato sauce; bring to a boil, scraping up any brown bits from pan. Reduce heat to low, cover and simmer, stirring occasionally, for about 45 minutes or until stew is thickened and juices run clear when chicken is pierced. Season to taste with salt and pepper.

Nutrients Per Serving	
Calories	190
Carbohydrate	5 g
Fiber	2 g
Protein	29 g
Fat	6 g
Iron	3 mg
Calcium	33 mg

Chicken, Cranberry and Mango Salad

Makes 4 servings

Whenever Theresa can, she adds cranberries to her meals for their health benefits. Combined with mango in this salad, the taste is divine. With the addition of chicken and rice, you have a complete, satisfying meal and an easy way to feed the family.

Tip

Look for a blend of whole-grain brown and Japanese black rice or use your favorite rice blend. When buying rice mixes, check the label carefully to make sure there are no gluten-containing grains added to the blend.

2 cups	reduced-sodium GF vegetable broth	500 mL
1 cup	GF brown and black rice blend	250 mL
1 cup	chopped cooked chicken or turkey	250 mL
1/2 cup	dried cranberries	125 mL
1/2 cup	chopped mango	125 mL
1/3 cup	slivered almonds	75 mL
1/4 cup	chopped green onions	60 mL
1 tsp	freshly squeezed lemon juice	5 mL
2 tbsp	extra virgin olive oil	30 mL
1 tbsp	brown or natural rice vinegar	15 mL
1 tbsp	chopped fresh basil	15 mL
	Salt and freshly ground black pepper	

1. In a large saucepan, combine broth and rice. Bring to a boil over high heat. Reduce heat to low, cover and simmer for 50 minutes or according to package directions, until rice is tender and liquid is absorbed.

2. In a large bowl, combine chicken, cranberries, mango, almonds and green onions. Sprinkle with lemon juice.

3. In a small bowl, whisk together oil, vinegar and basil. Drizzle over salad and toss to coat. Season to taste with salt and pepper.

4. Spread rice in a serving dish and arrange salad on top.

Nutrients Per Serving	
Calories	430
Carbohydrate	58 g
Fiber	5 g
Protein	17 g
Fat	14 g
Iron	2 mg
Calcium	32 mg

Chicken Pot Pie

Any combination of vegetables will work in this comforting, nutritious one-dish meal, so use whatever you have on hand, keeping the total amount to about 6 cups (1.5 L).

Tip

Choose your favorite GF non-dairy milk, such as soy, rice, almond or potato-based milk or, if you tolerate lactose, use regular 1% milk.

- Preheat oven to 350°F (180°C)
- 9-inch (23 cm) deep-dish glass pie plate, lightly greased

1 tsp	grapeseed oil	5 mL
1 tsp	butter	5 mL
8	boneless skinless chicken thighs (or 4 boneless skinless chicken breasts), cut into bite-size pieces	8
1	clove garlic, minced	1
1 cup	chopped onion	250 mL
1 cup	chopped red bell pepper	250 mL
1 cup	chopped celery	250 mL
1 cup	chopped carrots	250 mL
1 cup	chopped broccoli	250 mL
1 cup	frozen peas	250 mL
1/4 tsp	cayenne pepper	1 mL
1/4 tsp	dried tarragon	1 mL
1/4 tsp	dried Italian seasoning	1 mL
1 tbsp	white rice flour	15 mL
1 cup	fortified GF non-dairy milk or lactose-free 1% milk	250 mL
1 cup	shredded part-skim mozzarella cheese or mozzarella-style rice cheese	250 mL
	Salt and freshly ground black pepper	
	Pie Pastry for one 9-inch (23 cm) single-crust pie (see recipe, page 250)	

1. In a large saucepan, heat oil and butter over medium-high heat. Cook chicken for 5 to 7 minutes per side or until browned on both sides. Using a slotted spoon, transfer to a plate.

2. Reduce heat to medium. Add garlic, onion, red pepper, celery, carrots, broccoli, peas, cayenne, tarragon and Italian seasoning; sauté for 3 to 4 minutes or until softened. Sprinkle with flour and cook, stirring, for 1 minute. Gradually stir in milk.

3. Return chicken and any accumulated juices to pan. Reduce heat to medium-low and simmer, stirring often, for 10 to 12 minutes or until juices run clear when chicken is pierced and sauce is thickened.

Nutrients Per Serving	
Calories	400
Carbohydrate	33 g
Fiber	5 g
Protein	30 g
Fat	16 g
Iron	3 mg
Calcium	245 mg

Variation

Instead of covering the baking dish with pie pastry, spread 2 cups (500 mL) mashed potatoes or sweet potatoes thinly over the filling before baking.

Remove from heat and stir in cheese until melted. Season to taste with salt and pepper.

4. Transfer to prepared pie plate. Place pastry on top and press to seal edges. Trim off any excess pastry. Cut a few slits in the top to vent steam.

5. Bake in preheated oven for 20 minutes or until filling is bubbling and pastry is golden.

Grilled Chicken Kabobs

For this recipe, Theresa likes to put the chicken in the fridge to marinate first thing in the morning. Then, at suppertime, all she has to do is thread the chicken onto skewers and grill the kabobs. Serve with tzatziki on the side, as well as Quinoa Salad (page 183) or Greek Salad (page 180).

- Four 8- or 9-inch (20 or 23 cm) metal or wooden skewers

2 to 3	cloves garlic, minced	2 to 3
1½ tbsp	olive oil	22 mL
1 tsp	dried parsley	5 mL
½ tsp	dried oregano	2 mL
1 lb	boneless skinless chicken breasts, cut into 1½-inch (4 cm) cubes	500 g
	Salt and freshly ground black pepper	

1. In a large sealable plastic bag, combine garlic to taste, oil, parsley and oregano. Add chicken, seal and toss to coat. Refrigerate for at least 6 hours or overnight.

2. Preheat barbecue grill to medium. If using wooden skewers, soak them in water for 10 minutes.

3. Remove chicken from marinade, discarding marinade. Thread chicken onto skewers, leaving space between pieces. Grill chicken, turning often, for 7 to 10 minutes per side or until chicken is no longer pink inside. Season to taste with salt and pepper.

Oven-Baked Chicken Kabobs

To bake these kabobs instead of grilling them, place them on a rimmed baking sheet lined with parchment paper and bake in a 350°F (180°C) oven, turning once, for 20 minutes or until chicken is no longer pink inside.

Nutrients Per Serving

Calories	180
Carbohydrate	1 g
Fiber	0 g
Protein	26 g
Fat	7 g
Iron	1 mg
Calcium	19 mg

Turkey Fingers

Makes 4 servings

Turkey is a nice change from chicken, and it's available year-round in grocery stores, not just during the holiday season. These turkey fingers are particularly good with Sweet Potato Fries (page 234).

Tips

For added fiber and nutrients, try using GF multigrain crackers, such as Mary's Gone Crackers. Use your flavor of choice.

To crush the crackers, place them in a sealable plastic bag. Seal and use a rolling pin to crush them to the consistency of dry bread crumbs. Alternatively, you can crush them in a blender.

- Preheat oven to 350°F (180°C)
- Rimmed baking sheet, lined with parchment paper

1	egg	1
	Salt and freshly ground black pepper	
1/2 cup	GF cracker crumbs or bread crumbs	125 mL
1 tbsp	grated Romano cheese	15 mL
1/4 tsp	dried marjoram	1 mL
1/4 tsp	dried basil	1 mL
1/4 tsp	cayenne pepper	1 mL
1 lb	turkey breast scaloppini, cut into strips	500 g

1. In a bowl, lightly beat egg. Season with salt and pepper.

2. In a shallow dish, combine cracker crumbs, cheese, marjoram, basil and cayenne.

3. Dip turkey strips in egg mixture, then press in crumb mixture, coating lightly and shaking off excess. Place turkey on prepared baking sheet. Discard any excess egg mixture and crumb mixture.

4. Bake in preheated oven for 20 minutes or until coating is golden brown and turkey is no longer pink inside.

Nutrients Per Serving

Calories	210
Carbohydrate	10 g
Fiber	1 g
Protein	31 g
Fat	4.5 g
Iron	2 mg
Calcium	43 mg

Turkey Sausage with Lima Bean Medley

This divine medley of lima beans, broccoli and mushrooms becomes even more scrumptious when turkey sausage is added to the mix. Serve over cooked brown rice and enjoy a glass of red wine with your meal.

2 tbsp	grapeseed oil	30 mL
1 lb	turkey sausages (about 4), removed from casings	500 g
1 cup	sliced mushrooms	250 mL
1/2 cup	chopped onion	125 mL
1 cup	frozen chopped broccoli	250 mL
1 cup	frozen lima beans	250 mL
1 tbsp	chopped fresh parsley	15 mL
1 tbsp	red wine vinegar	15 mL
	Salt and freshly ground black pepper	

1. In a large skillet, heat oil over medium heat. Cook sausage, breaking it up with the back of a spoon, for 7 to 10 minutes or until no longer pink. Using a slotted spoon, transfer to a plate lined with paper towels.

2. Add mushrooms and onion to skillet; sauté for about 5 minutes or until mushrooms are browned and crisp. Add broccoli, beans, parsley and vinegar; sauté for 5 to 8 minutes or until tender. Return sausage to skillet and simmer, stirring, until heated through. Season to taste with salt and pepper.

Nutrients Per Serving

Calories	280
Carbohydrate	16 g
Fiber	4 g
Protein	19 g
Fat	16 g
Iron	3 mg
Calcium	58 mg

Three-Bean Chili with Turkey

There are so many wonderful options when it comes to beans that it's seems a shame to make chili from just one kind. So this tasty turkey chili contains three of Theresa's favorites.

Tips

After emptying the tomatoes from the can, rinse the can with the water (the amount of water specified in step 2 is one full can) before adding it to the pan, to capture all the juices that cling to the sides.

A 19-oz (540 mL) can of beans will yield about 2 cups (500 mL) once the beans are drained and rinsed. If you have smaller or larger cans, you can use the volume called for or just add the amount from your can.

Instead of the cumin and coriander, you can use 1 tsp (5 mL) GF chili powder.

Nutrients Per Serving

Calories	260
Carbohydrate	33 g
Fiber	11 g
Protein	21 g
Fat	6 g
Iron	4 mg
Calcium	105 mg

1 tsp	grapeseed oil	5 mL
1 lb	lean ground turkey	500 g
1	clove garlic, minced	1
1 cup	chopped onion	250 mL
1 cup	chopped celery	250 mL
1 cup	chopped carrots	250 mL
1	can (28 oz/796 mL) crushed tomatoes (see tip, at left)	1
2 cups	rinsed drained canned romano beans	500 mL
2 cups	rinsed drained canned black beans	500 mL
2 cups	rinsed drained canned lentils	500 mL
1 tsp	dried oregano	5 mL
1 tsp	cayenne pepper	5 mL
$\frac{1}{2}$ tsp	ground cumin	2 mL
$\frac{1}{2}$ tsp	ground coriander	2 mL
$\frac{1}{4}$ tsp	salt	1 mL

1. In a large saucepan, heat oil over medium-high heat. Cook turkey, breaking it up with the back of a spoon, for about 7 minutes or until no longer pink. Add garlic, onion, celery and carrots; sauté for 3 to 4 minutes or until tender.

2. Stir in tomatoes, $3\frac{1}{4}$ cups (800 mL) water, romano beans, black beans, lentils, oregano, cayenne, cumin, coriander and salt; bring to a boil. Cover, leaving lid ajar, reduce heat to low and simmer, stirring occasionally, for $1\frac{1}{2}$ hours to blend the flavors.

Side Dishes

Stuffed Artichokes

Makes 4 servings

Not only are artichokes a great source of iron, but they're also a great deal of fun to eat. Peel off one petal, place it between your teeth and pull, leaving the tender part in your mouth and discarding the unwanted leaf. When you reach the center, discard the choke and enjoy the tender base.

Tip

The cooking time depends on the size of the artichoke. When choosing your artichokes, make sure they are all the same size, so they'll all be done at the same time. Theresa prefers small artichokes.

8	small artichokes (about 1 lb/500 g)	8
	Lemon wedges	
½ cup	GF cracker crumbs	125 mL
2 to 3	cloves garlic, minced	2 to 3
2 tsp	dried parsley	10 mL
	Salt and freshly ground black pepper	
2 tbsp	olive oil	30 mL

1. Cut the stems off the artichokes, creating a flat base. Trim off the tough outer leaves. Cut about ½ inch (1 cm) off the tops, then use scissors to snip off the sharp leaf tips. Push open the leaves and rinse. Rub all cut surfaces with lemon.

2. In a small bowl, combine cracker crumbs, garlic to taste and parsley. Season with salt and pepper to taste. Stir in oil to make a paste.

3. Stuff artichokes with cracker mixture and place upright in a large pot. Add enough water to come halfway up artichokes. Cover and bring to a boil over high heat. Reduce heat to low and simmer for 45 minutes or until tender.

Nutrients Per Serving	
Calories	180
Carbohydrate	22 g
Fiber	8 g
Protein	5 g
Fat	9 g
Iron	2 mg
Calcium	74 mg

Asparagus Wraps

Makes 2 to 4 servings

Theresa's oldest brother, Louis, gets all the credit for creating this simple, delicious side dish.

Nutrients Per Serving	
Calories	190
Carbohydrate	4 g
Fiber	1 g
Protein	5 g
Fat	13 g
Iron	0.5 mg
Calcium	217 mg

- Preheat oven to 300°F (150°C)
- Rimmed baking sheet, lined with parchment paper

4	slices prosciutto	4
12	spears asparagus, ends trimmed	12
4	thin strips red bell pepper	4
4	thin slices part-skim mozzarella cheese	4
2 tbsp	olive oil	30 mL

1. Lay prosciutto out on a work surface. Place 3 asparagus spears, 1 red pepper strip and 1 mozzarella slice in the center of each prosciutto slice and wrap prosciutto around the filling. Place on prepared baking sheet and brush with oil.

2. Bake in preheated oven for 20 minutes or until asparagus is tender.

Fennel and Sun-Dried Tomatoes

Makes 2 servings

Sautéed fennel has a very mild licorice flavor and is delicious on its own or served over rice.

Nutrients Per Serving	
Calories	160
Carbohydrate	20 g
Fiber	8 g
Protein	4 g
Fat	9 g
Iron	2 mg
Calcium	119 mg

1 tbsp	grapeseed oil	15 mL
1	fennel bulb, trimmed and cut into $\frac{1}{4}$-inch (0.5 cm) thick slices	1
$\frac{1}{4}$ cup	sliced drained oil-packed sun-dried tomatoes	60 mL
1 tbsp	chopped fresh parsley	15 mL
	Salt and freshly ground black pepper	

1. In a skillet, heat oil over medium heat. Sauté fennel for 5 to 7 minutes or until tender and golden brown. Add sun-dried tomatoes and parsley; sauté for 1 minute. Season to taste with salt and pepper.

Green Beans and Romano Cheese

Makes 4 servings

This delicious side is a great way to get kids to eat their vegetables. Serve it alongside steak, chicken or pasta dishes.

Tip

If you use fresh green beans instead of frozen, blanch them in a pot of boiling water for 3 minutes first.

Variation

Substitute fresh or frozen broccoli for the beans. If using fresh, blanch it first.

2 tbsp	grapeseed oil	30 mL
3 to 4	cloves garlic, minced	3 to 4
4 cups	frozen cut green beans	1 L
2 tbsp	chopped fresh parsley	30 mL
1/4 cup	grated Romano cheese	60 mL
	Freshly ground black pepper	

1. In a skillet, heat oil over medium heat. Sauté garlic to taste, green beans and parsley for 12 to 15 minutes or until beans are tender-crisp. Stir in cheese. Season to taste with pepper.

Nutrients Per Serving	
Calories	160
Carbohydrate	10 g
Fiber	3 g
Protein	6 g
Fat	11 g
Iron	1 mg
Calcium	233 mg

Peas and Mushrooms

This side dish is served at just about every Italian party, often with Fatina (page 213), but there's no reason to wait for a celebration — enjoy it any night of the week!

Nutrients Per Serving	
Calories	150
Carbohydrate	16 g
Fiber	5 g
Protein	6 g
Fat	7 g
Iron	2 mg
Calcium	34 mg

2 tbsp	olive or grapeseed oil	30 mL
8 oz	mushrooms, sliced	250 g
½ cup	chopped onion	125 mL
2 cups	frozen peas	500 mL
	Salt and freshly ground black pepper	

1. In a skillet, heat oil over medium-high heat. Sauté mushrooms and onion for 5 to 7 minutes or until browned. Add peas and sauté for 5 to 7 minutes or until heated through. Season to taste with salt and pepper.

Spinach with Almonds

Did you know that cooked spinach has more iron than raw spinach? And you can up the iron even more by topping it off with almonds.

Nutrients Per Serving	
Calories	140
Carbohydrate	5 g
Fiber	3 g
Protein	5 g
Fat	12 g
Iron	2 mg
Calcium	106 mg

1	package (10 oz/300 g) fresh spinach, trimmed	1
2 tbsp	olive oil	30 mL
½ cup	slivered almonds	125 mL
	Salt and freshly ground black pepper	

1. Rinse spinach under cold running water. In a large saucepan, over medium-high heat, cook spinach in the water clinging to the leaves, stirring, for 3 to 5 minutes or until wilted. Drain and transfer to a serving platter.

2. Drizzle oil over spinach and sprinkle with almonds. Season to taste with salt and pepper.

Rapini, Red Pepper and Sun-Dried Tomatoes

Makes 4 servings

Rapini, also called broccoli rabe, is a source of vitamin A, vitamin C, potassium, calcium and iron. In this recipe, its bitter flavor is tempered by the sweetness of the red pepper.

1	bunch rapini (about 1 lb/500 g), trimmed and cut into bite-size pieces	1
2 tbsp	grapeseed oil	30 mL
1 cup	chopped red bell pepper	250 mL
½ cup	sliced drained oil-packed sun-dried tomatoes	125 mL
	Salt and freshly ground black pepper	

1. Place rapini in a large pot and add enough water to cover. Bring to a boil over high heat. Drain.

2. In a skillet, heat oil over medium-high heat. Sauté rapini for 1 minute. Add red pepper and sauté for 5 to 7 minutes or until tender. Add sun-dried tomatoes and sauté for 1 minute. Season to taste with salt and pepper.

Nutrients Per Serving	
Calories	130
Carbohydrate	11 g
Fiber	2 g
Protein	5 g
Fat	9 g
Iron	2 mg
Calcium	62 mg

Pizza Topping Stir-Fry

Makes 2 servings

This fun stir-fry contains all the best vegetarian pizza toppings (in Theresa's opinion). Eat it as is or serve it over cooked wild rice or GF pasta.

2 tsp	grapeseed oil	10 mL
1½ cups	chopped eggplant	375 mL
1 cup	chopped red bell pepper	250 mL
¼ cup	chopped onion	60 mL
⅓ cup	quartered drained marinated artichoke hearts	75 mL
¼ cup	sliced drained oil-packed sun-dried tomatoes	60 mL
¼ cup	sliced green olives stuffed with pimentos	60 mL
	Freshly ground black pepper	

1. In a saucepan, heat oil over medium-high heat. Sauté eggplant, red pepper and onion for 5 to 7 minutes or until softened. Add artichokes, sun-dried tomatoes and olives; sauté for 1 minute or until heated through. Season to taste with pepper.

Nutrients Per Serving	
Calories	190
Carbohydrate	15 g
Fiber	5 g
Protein	3 g
Fat	15 g
Iron	1 mg
Calcium	37 mg

Stuffed Zucchini

Zucchini, a variety of summer squash, has a light, delicate flavor that is enhanced by the garlic-and-herb stuffing in this recipe. (And the stuffing is delicious with tomatoes, too!)

Variation

Substitute 2 large tomatoes for the zucchini and cook for 20 to 30 minutes or until tomatoes are tender.

- Preheat oven to 350°F (180°C)
- 8-inch (20 cm) square glass baking dish, lightly greased

2	zucchini	2
1	clove garlic, minced	1
¼ cup	GF dry bread crumbs or cracker crumbs	60 mL
1 tbsp	chopped fresh parsley	15 mL
2 tsp	olive oil	10 mL
	Salt and freshly ground black pepper	

1. Cut off ends of zucchini, then cut zucchini in half lengthwise. Using a spoon, remove some of the flesh from the center of each zucchini half. Place cut side up in prepared baking dish.

2. In a small bowl, combine garlic, bread crumbs, parsley and oil. Season to taste with salt and pepper. Spread evenly in hollowed-out zucchini.

3. Cover and bake in preheated oven for 20 to 30 minutes or until zucchini are tender.

Nutrients Per Serving	
Calories	60
Carbohydrate	7 g
Fiber	1 g
Protein	1 g
Fat	3.5 g
Iron	0.5 mg
Calcium	21 mg

Sage Chips

Makes 2 to 4 servings

This recipe is pure simplicity, but it's amazing how delicious sage chips are alongside Meatloaf (page 216), Chicken Pot Pie (page 220) or Turkey Fingers (page 222). You can make these on the stovetop while the main course is in the oven. They're great as a snack, too!

Variation

Substitute twenty-four ⅛-inch (3 mm) thick round zucchini slices for the sage leaves and increase the cooking time to 1 to 2 minutes per side.

1	egg	1
2 tbsp	sorghum flour	30 mL
	Salt and freshly ground black pepper	
24	fresh sage leaves	24
2 tbsp	grapeseed oil	30 mL

1. In a small bowl, whisk together egg and flour until well combined. Season with salt and pepper.

2. Working with 12 sage leaves at a time, dip leaves in egg mixture, coating both sides. In a skillet, heat oil over medium heat. Cook sage leaves for about 1 minute per side or until golden brown. Using tongs, transfer to a plate lined with paper towels. Repeat with the remaining sage.

Nutrients Per Serving	
Calories	100
Carbohydrate	5 g
Fiber	0 g
Protein	2 g
Fat	9 g
Iron	0.4 mg
Calcium	53 mg

Sweet Potato Fries

Who doesn't love fries? And when you sub in sweet potatoes for the potatoes and bake them instead of frying, fries actually become good for you as well as delicious!

- Preheat oven to 350°F (180°C)
- Rimmed baking sheet, lined with parchment paper

1 lb	sweet potatoes, peeled and cut into ¼-inch (0.5 cm) thick slices	500 g
2 tsp	grapeseed oil	10 mL
2 tbsp	grated Romano cheese	30 mL
	Salt and freshly ground black pepper	

1. In a large bowl, toss sweet potatoes, oil and cheese until sweet potatoes are well coated. Spread out in a single layer on prepared baking sheet.

2. Bake in preheated oven for 20 to 30 minutes, turning halfway through, until crispy and golden. Season to taste with salt and pepper.

Nutrients Per Serving

Calories	120
Carbohydrate	20 g
Fiber	3 g
Protein	3 g
Fat	3 g
Iron	1 mg
Calcium	61 mg

Potato and Sweet Potato Bake

Makes 4 servings

Baked potatoes: good. Baked sweet potatoes: good. Baked potatoes *and* sweet potatoes? Awesome. This dish is a great accompaniment to Fatina (page 213) or Grilled Chicken Kabobs (page 221).

- Preheat oven to 350°F (180°C)
- 13- by 9-inch (23 by 23 cm) glass baking dish

8 oz	potatoes, cut into 1-inch (2.5 cm) cubes	250 g
8 oz	sweet potato, cut into 1-inch (2.5 cm) cubes	250 g
¼ cup	raisins	60 mL
1 tbsp	olive oil	15 mL
1 tbsp	melted butter	15 mL
1 tsp	dried rosemary	5 mL
	Salt and freshly ground black pepper	

1. In baking dish, combine potatoes, sweet potatoes and raisins. Add oil, butter, rosemary and salt and pepper to taste; toss to coat.

2. Cover and bake in preheated oven for 20 minutes. Uncover and bake for 20 to 25 minutes or until potatoes are tender and crispy.

Nutrients Per Serving

Calories	120
Carbohydrate	19 g
Fiber	2 g
Protein	2 g
Fat	4 g
Iron	1 mg
Calcium	16 mg

Gnocchi

Makes 7 servings

Making gnocchi was a
Sunday morning ritual in
Theresa's family. Now, with
this gluten-free version,
you can make your own
family memories.

Tip

To cook gnocchi, add to a
pot of boiling salted water
and cook, gently stirring,
for 2 to 3 minutes (or about
5 minutes from frozen), until
all gnocchi rise to the top.
Drain, toss with spaghetti
sauce and serve sprinkled
with grated Romano
cheese.

Nutrients Per Serving	
Calories	290
Carbohydrate	61 g
Fiber	3 g
Protein	6 g
Fat	2 g
Iron	1 mg
Calcium	25 mg

- Stand mixer with dough hook
- Baking sheets, lightly dusted with white rice flour

2 lbs	oblong baking potatoes, such as russet (about 4)	1 kg
3	eggs	3
¾ cup	potato starch	175 mL
¾ cup	potato flour	175 mL
½ cup	white rice flour (approx.)	125 mL

1. Place potatoes in a large pot and add enough water to cover. Bring to a boil over high heat. Reduce heat and simmer for 30 to 45 minutes or until potato skins break and potatoes are tender. Drain.

2. Peel skin off potatoes, place potatoes in bowl of stand mixer and mash with a potato masher. Using the mixer with the dough hook attached, beat in eggs, one at a time, on low speed. Gradually mix in potato starch and potato flour, mixing until dough pulls away from the sides of the bowl. Beat in about ½ cup (125 mL) water, 1 tbsp (15 mL) at a time, until dough is soft and pliable but not sticky. Divide dough into 16 equal portions.

3. Sprinkle a cutting board with rice flour. Working with one portion of dough at a time, roll it under your hands into a long, thin rope, about 12 inches (30 cm) long and ½ inch (1 cm) thick, keeping your hands and the board well floured. Using a sharp knife, cut rope on a slight angle into ½-inch (1 cm) pieces. Sprinkle dough pieces with rice flour and place on prepared baking sheet. Repeat until all the dough is cut into gnocchi. Slide the baking sheet back and forth to ensure that all the pieces are covered in flour.

4. Cook immediately or cover with a sheet of parchment paper and freeze until solid. Once frozen, transfer to a sealable freezer bag and freeze for up to 3 months.

Nokedli

Nokedli are small flour dumplings made with a spaetzle maker (available at kitchen stores). This gluten-free version was inspired by Theresa's friend Janice's recipe.

Tip

To serve nokedli, divide the dumplings among bowls and ladle stew, such as Veal Stew (page 217), over top. Or, for a really fast meal, simply ladle spaghetti sauce over top and sprinkle with grated Romano cheese.

- Spaetzle maker

1 cup	sorghum flour	250 mL
1 cup	white rice flour	250 mL
½ cup	potato starch	125 mL
½ tsp	salt	2 mL
2	eggs	2
1 cup	cold water	250 mL

1. In a bowl, whisk together sorghum flour, rice flour, potato starch and salt.

2. In a large bowl, whisk together eggs and cold water. Using a wooden spoon, stir in dry ingredients until smooth.

3. In a large pot, bring 12 cups (3 L) water to a boil over high heat. Reduce heat to medium and lay spaetzle maker across top of pot. Fill spaetzle maker with 1 cup (250 mL) batter, sliding the handle back and forth so that all the batter falls through into the water. Repeat until the batter is used up. Boil for 1 to 2 minutes or until nokedli float to the top. Drain.

Nutrients Per Serving	
Calories	230
Carbohydrate	46 g
Fiber	3 g
Protein	6 g
Fat	3 g
Iron	1 mg
Calcium	7 mg

Quinoa Pesto Pilaf

Quinoa is delicious and versatile, not to mention nutritious! Alexandra's daughter, Brooke, loves this side dish (she calls it "couscous"). Serve it alongside barbecued fish or chicken drumsticks with corn on the cob. Or try it with Grilled Chicken Kabobs (page 221) and Greek Salad (page 180).

1 cup	quinoa, rinsed	250 mL
1 cup	chopped drained oil-packed sun-dried tomatoes	250 mL
3 tbsp	basil pesto	45 mL
1 tbsp	olive oil	15 mL
	Freshly ground black pepper	

1. In a saucepan, bring 2 cups (500 mL) water to a boil over high heat. Add quinoa, reduce heat to low, cover and simmer for 20 minutes or until quinoa is tender and liquid is almost absorbed. Remove from heat and let stand, covered, for 5 minutes or until liquid is absorbed.

2. Using a fork, gently stir in sun-dried tomatoes, pesto and oil. Season to taste with pepper.

Nutrients Per Serving

Calories	250
Carbohydrate	31 g
Fiber	5 g
Protein	8 g
Fat	11 g
Iron	3 mg
Calcium	85 mg

Snacks and Desserts

Hot Spinach and Broccoli Dip

Whenever Theresa serves this dip, it's gone within 20 minutes. It's fabulous hot or cold (if you have any left). Serve it with crudités, GF crackers, GF corn chips or potato chips.

- Preheat oven to 350°F (180°C)
- 8-inch (20 cm) round metal baking pan, lightly greased

1 cup	chopped fresh spinach	250 mL
½ cup	finely chopped broccoli	125 mL
¼ cup	chopped red onion	60 mL
¼ cup	chopped red bell pepper	60 mL
3	cloves garlic, minced (optional)	3
1 cup	shredded reduced-fat Cheddar cheese or Cheddar-style rice cheese	250 mL
¼ cup	grated Romano cheese	60 mL
¾ cup	plain low-fat yogurt or soy yogurt	175 mL
¼ cup	light GF mayonnaise	60 mL

1. In a large bowl, combine spinach, broccoli, red onion, red pepper and garlic (if using). Stir in Cheddar, Romano, yogurt and mayonnaise. Spread evenly in prepared pan.

2. Bake in preheated oven for 30 to 40 minutes or until cheese is golden and bubbly. Let cool for 10 to 15 minutes, then transfer to a serving dish.

Nutrients Per Serving

Calories	80
Carbohydrate	4 g
Fiber	1 g
Protein	6 g
Fat	5 g
Iron	0.2 mg
Calcium	129 mg

White Bean Dip

This dip is a tasty alternative to hummus. It is cost-effective, takes minutes to prepare and is low-fat and nutritious. Pack it along for an on-the-go snack with gluten-free multigrain crackers or baby carrots.

Tips

A 19-oz (540 mL) can of beans will yield about 2 cups (500 mL) once the beans are drained and rinsed. If you have smaller or larger cans, you can use the volume called for or just add the amount from your can. If you're soaking and cooking dried beans, you'll need 1 cup (250 mL).

Tahini is a paste made from sesame seeds. It is available in the international foods section of supermarkets and at natural food stores. The oil from the paste tends to float to the top of the jar, so give it a good stir before you measure it.

Nutrients Per Serving

Calories	110
Carbohydrate	15 g
Fiber	3 g
Protein	5 g
Fat	3 g
Iron	2 mg
Calcium	54 mg

• Food processor

2 cups	cooked or canned white kidney beans, drained and rinsed	500 mL
1 tsp	paprika	5 mL
1 tsp	ground cumin	5 mL
1/2 tsp	garlic powder	2 mL
1/4 tsp	salt	1 mL
1/4 tsp	freshly ground black pepper	1 mL
2 tbsp	freshly squeezed lemon juice	30 mL
1 tbsp	olive oil	15 mL
1 tbsp	tahini (see tip, at left)	15 mL

1. In a food processor fitted with a metal blade, combine beans, paprika, cumin, garlic powder, salt, pepper, lemon juice, oil and tahini. Pulse until smooth, adding water 2 tbsp (30 mL) at a time until dip is desired consistency.

2. Serve immediately or transfer to an airtight container and refrigerate for up to 1 week.

Trail Mix

Makes 3½ cups
(875 mL)
(¼ cup/60 mL
per serving)

Start with this basic recipe and sub in other ingredients depending on what strikes your fancy and what you have on hand. Good additions include raisins, shredded coconut, hazelnuts and even chunks of dark chocolate. Be creative — trail mix can be a little different every time you make it!

½ cup	dried apricots, cut into quarters	125 mL
½ cup	dried cranberries	125 mL
½ cup	dried goji berries (optional)	125 mL
½ cup	whole almonds	125 mL
½ cup	chopped walnuts	125 mL
½ cup	unsalted sunflower seeds	125 mL
½ cup	raw green pumpkin seeds (pepitas)	125 mL

1. In a large bowl, combine apricots, cranberries, goji berries (if using), almonds, walnuts, sunflower seeds and pumpkin seeds.

2. Store in an airtight container at room temperature for up 1 month.

Nutrients Per Serving	
Calories	150
Carbohydrate	10 g
Fiber	2 g
Protein	4 g
Fat	11 g
Iron	1 mg
Calcium	24 mg

Almond Cookies

Makes 24 to 30 cookies (1 per serving)

This recipe comes to us from Joni Frydrych of Joni's Kitchen. Joni is the vice-president of the Toronto chapter of the Canadian Celiac Association and has been cooking and baking gluten-free ever since her daughter, Haley, was diagnosed with celiac disease.

Tip

For a nice presentation, dip one end of cooled cookies into melted GF chocolate.

- Preheat oven to 350°F (180°C)
- Food processor
- Baking sheets, lined with parchment paper

2½ cups	ground almonds	625 mL
1 cup	granulated sugar	250 mL
1 tsp	almond or vanilla extract	5 mL
3	egg whites	3

1. In food processor fitted with a metal blade, process almonds and sugar until blended. Add almond extract and egg whites; process until a firm paste forms.

2. Scoop about 1 tbsp (15 mL) of dough and shape into a ball, then pinch into a quarter-moon shape. Place cookies 1 inch (2.5 cm) apart on prepared baking sheets.

3. Bake, one sheet at a time, in preheated oven for 10 to 12 minutes or until golden but still soft. Let cool on baking sheets on a wire rack for 2 minutes, then transfer to the rack to cool.

Nutrients Per Serving	
Calories	60
Carbohydrate	7 g
Fiber	1 g
Protein	2 g
Fat	4 g
Iron	0.3 mg
Calcium	21 mg

Chocolate Chip Cookies

Theresa has been baking these cookies for over 15 years, and they are fantastic each and every time. Young or old, everyone loves a chocolate chip cookie.

Tip

Store these cookies in a cookie tin or canister at room temperature for up to 5 days.

- Preheated oven 350°F (180°C)
- Rimmed baking sheets, lined with parchment paper

½ cup	white rice flour	125 mL
½ cup	brown rice flour	125 mL
1 tsp	baking soda	5 mL
¼ tsp	salt	1 mL
¾ cup	granulated raw cane sugar	175 mL
½ cup	butter, softened	125 mL
2	eggs	2
2 tsp	vanilla extract	10 mL
1 cup	GF semisweet chocolate chips	250 mL

1. In a small bowl, whisk together white rice flour, brown rice flour, baking soda and salt.

2. In a large bowl, using an electric mixer, cream sugar and butter. Beat in eggs, one at a time, and vanilla until well blended. Stir in flour mixture until combined. Stir in chocolate chips.

3. Drop dough by rounded spoonfuls about 2 inches (5 cm) apart on prepared baking sheets. Flatten slightly with a fork.

4. Bake, one sheet at a time, in preheated oven for 8 to 10 minutes or until edges are slightly browned and centers are set. Let cool on baking sheets on a wire rack for 2 minutes, then transfer to the rack to cool.

Nutrients Per Serving	
Calories	120
Carbohydrate	15 g
Fiber	1 g
Protein	1 g
Fat	6 g
Iron	0.3 mg
Calcium	5 mg

Hazelnut Shortbread

Theresa's sister Susan makes the best shortbread. Here's a gluten-free version of her recipe.

Tips

The dough can be stored in the refrigerator for up to 3 days or in the freezer for up to 1 month.

For an extra-special treat, dip cooled cookies in melted GF chocolate and sprinkle with ground hazelnuts.

- Baking sheets, lined with parchment paper

1 cup	white rice flour	250 mL
½ cup	sorghum flour	125 mL
⅓ cup	ground hazelnuts	75 mL
Pinch	salt	Pinch
½ cup	granulated raw cane sugar	125 mL
1 cup	butter, softened	250 mL
1	egg	1
½ tsp	vanilla extract	2 mL

1. In a medium bowl, whisk together white rice flour, sorghum flour, hazelnuts and salt.

2. In a large bowl, using an electric mixer, cream sugar and butter until light and fluffy. Beat in egg and vanilla until well blended. Stir in flour mixture until combined.

3. Divide dough in half. Place half the dough on a sheet of parchment paper and roll it under your hands into a 1-inch (2.5 cm) thick log. Repeat with the remaining dough. Wrap both logs in plastic wrap and refrigerate for 30 minutes or until firm. Meanwhile, preheat oven to 325°F (160°C).

4. Slice dough into ¼-inch (0.5 cm) slices. Place 1 inch (2.5 cm) apart on prepared baking sheets.

5. Bake, one sheet at a time, for 12 to 15 minutes or until edges are golden brown. Transfer cookies to a wire rack and let cool completely.

Nutrients Per Serving

Calories	50
Carbohydrate	4 g
Fiber	0 g
Protein	0 g
Fat	4 g
Iron	0 mg
Calcium	2 mg

Cranberry Clusters

These festive cookies are a great choice for a cookie exchange during the holiday season, but they're delicious at any time of year!

Tip

Store these cookies in a cookie tin or canister at room temperature for up to 5 days.

- Preheat oven to 375°F (190°C)
- Baking sheets, lined with parchment paper

¾ cup	white rice flour	175 mL
¼ tsp	baking soda	1 mL
¼ cup	granulated raw cane sugar	60 mL
¼ cup	butter, softened	60 mL
2	eggs	2
1 cup	dried cranberries	250 mL
½ cup	GF semisweet chocolate chips	125 mL
½ cup	chopped walnuts	125 mL

1. In a small bowl, combine white rice flour and baking soda.

2. In a large bowl, using an electric mixer, cream sugar and butter until light and fluffy. Beat in eggs, one at a time, until well blended. Stir in flour mixture until combined. Stir in cranberries, chocolate chips and walnuts.

3. Drop dough by rounded spoonfuls 2 inches (5 cm) apart on prepared baking sheets. Flatten slightly with a fork.

4. Bake, one sheet at a time, in preheated oven for 8 to 10 minutes or until tops are golden and edges are set. Let cool on baking sheets on a wire rack for 2 minutes, then transfer to the rack to cool.

Nutrients Per Serving	
Calories	90
Carbohydrate	11 g
Fiber	1 g
Protein	1 g
Fat	5 g
Iron	0.3 mg
Calcium	22 mg

Chocolate Hazelnut Biscotti

In Italy, these twice-baked cookies are served in the morning with espresso or cappuccino. The hard cookies soften a bit when dipped in the coffee.

Tip

For special occasions, spread melted chocolate over cooled biscotti and sprinkle with finely chopped nuts.

Store biscotti in a cookie tin or canister at room temperature for up to 2 weeks.

- Preheat oven to 350°F (180°C)
- Baking sheets, lined with parchment paper

1 cup	brown rice flour	250 mL
2 tbsp	unsweetened cocoa powder	30 mL
2 tsp	GF baking powder	10 mL
1/4 tsp	salt	1 mL
1/2 cup	granulated raw cane sugar	125 mL
3	eggs	3
1/2 cup	chopped hazelnuts or walnuts	125 mL

1. In a small bowl, whisk together brown rice flour, cocoa, baking powder and salt.

2. In a large bowl, whisk together sugar and eggs until frothy. Stir in flour mixture until combined. Stir in hazelnuts. Let batter stand for 15 minutes to thicken. Stir batter.

3. Spoon batter into two rectangular mounds, each 9 by 4 inches (23 by 10 cm), about 2 inches (5 cm) apart on one prepared baking sheet. Bake in preheated oven for 15 to 20 minutes or until a tester inserted in the center comes out clean. Remove from oven, leaving oven on, and let cool for 10 minutes.

4. Using a serrated knife, cut mounds on the diagonal into 1/2-inch (1 cm) slices. Place slices cut side down on baking sheets.

5. Bake for 8 to 10 minutes or until tops are firm. Flip biscotti over and bake for 8 to 10 minutes or until firm and dry. Transfer to a rack and let cool completely.

Nutrients Per Serving	
Calories	40
Carbohydrate	6 g
Fiber	0 g
Protein	1 g
Fat	2 g
Iron	0.2 mg
Calcium	6 mg

Peanut Butter and Chocolate Rice Crisp Bars

**Makes 12 bars
(1 per serving)**

Theresa's son Joseph loves these treats, and no wonder — the combination of chocolate and peanut butter can't be beat!

Tip

Be sure to use unsalted, unsweetened peanut butter for this recipe.

Variation

Substitute cashew butter or hazelnut butter for the peanut butter.

- 8-inch (20 cm) square baking pan, lightly greased

1 cup	natural peanut butter	250 mL
1 cup	GF semisweet chocolate chips	250 mL
½ cup	agave nectar	125 mL
¼ tsp	salt	1 mL
4 cups	brown rice crisp cereal	1 L
1 tsp	vanilla extract	5 mL

1. In a large saucepan, over low heat, combine peanut butter, chocolate chips, agave nectar and salt. Cook, stirring, until melted and smooth.

2. Remove from heat and stir in cereal and vanilla until cereal is well coated. Press evenly into prepared baking pan. Refrigerate for 20 minutes or until firm. Cut into bars.

Nutrients Per Serving	
Calories	270
Carbohydrate	33 g
Fiber	3 g
Protein	7 g
Fat	15 g
Iron	1 mg
Calcium	17 mg

Chocolate Chip Brownies

If you love chocolate, you're going to love these brownies. Enjoy them with your friends and family — no one will know they're gluten-free!

- Preheat oven to 350°F (180°C)
- 8-inch (20 cm) square metal baking pan, lined with parchment paper, leaving a 2-inch (5 cm) overhang

¼ cup	sorghum flour	60 mL
¼ cup	tapioca starch	60 mL
¼ cup	unsweetened cocoa powder	60 mL
1 tsp	GF baking powder	5 mL
¼ tsp	salt	1 mL
¾ cup	granulated raw cane sugar	175 mL
¼ cup	sunflower oil	60 mL
¼ cup	unsweetened applesauce	60 mL
2	eggs	2
1 tsp	vanilla extract	5 mL
½ cup	GF semisweet chocolate chips	125 mL
1 cup	chopped walnuts (optional)	250 mL

Icing (optional)

½ cup	GF semisweet chocolate chips	125 mL

1. In a small bowl, whisk together sorghum flour, tapioca starch, cocoa, baking powder and salt.

2. In a large bowl, whisk together sugar, oil and applesauce. Beat in eggs, one at a time, and vanilla until well blended. Stir in flour mixture until just combined. Fold in chocolate chips and walnuts (if using). Spread evenly in prepared baking pan.

3. Bake in preheated oven for 35 to 40 minutes or until a tester inserted in the center comes out clean. Let cool completely in pan on a wire rack.

4. *Icing:* Meanwhile, if desired, place chocolate chips in a small saucepan. Place on the stovetop and let the heat from the oven melt the chocolate. Stir until smooth and spread over cooled brownies.

5. Let cool completely in pan on a rack. Using parchment paper as handles, transfer to a cutting board, then cut into squares.

Nutrients Per Serving	
Calories	120
Carbohydrate	17 g
Fiber	1 g
Protein	1 g
Fat	6 g
Iron	1 mg
Calcium	9 mg

Pie Pastry

This all-purpose pie pastry
works just as well for
savory recipes as it does
for sweet desserts.

Tips

We prefer to use a vegan
non-hydrogenated
shortening, such as Earth
Balance natural shortening.

To fit pastry into a pie plate,
remove the top sheet of
parchment and place a
greased pie plate upside
down on the pastry. Place
your hand under the bottom
sheet of parchment and flip
the pastry over, easing it
into the pie plate. Carefully
remove the parchment.

If your recipe instructs you
to partially bake the pie
pastry before filling it, prick
the bottom and sides with a
fork. Bake at 325°F (160°C)
for about 20 minutes or until
firm. Let cool completely
before filling.

Nutrients Per 1/6 pie	
Calories	140
Carbohydrate	18 g
Fiber	1 g
Protein	3 g
Fat	6 g
Iron	0.7 mg
Calcium	3 mg

3 cups	sorghum flour	750 mL
2½ cups	brown rice flour	625 mL
¾ cup	tapioca starch	175 mL
¼ cup	teff flour	60 mL
¼ cup	granulated raw cane sugar	60 mL
1 tsp	salt	5 mL
2 cups	cold vegetable shortening, cut into cubes (see tip, at left)	500 mL
2	eggs	2
1 tbsp	GF rice vinegar	15 mL
	Cold water	

For Each Pie Crust

1	egg white	1

1. In a very large bowl, combine sorghum flour, brown rice flour, tapioca starch, teff flour, sugar and salt. Using a pastry blender or two knives, cut in shortening until mixture resembles coarse crumbs. Set aside.

2. In a glass measuring cup, whisk together eggs and vinegar. Add enough cold water to measure 1 cup (250 mL). Using a wooden spoon, stir into flour mixture until starting to hold together.

3. Gather dough with your hands and divide into 7 equal portions (each about 8 oz/250 g), squeezing to shape into a ball. Use immediately or wrap in plastic wrap and store in the refrigerator for up to 2 days or in the freezer for up to 4 months. Thaw frozen pie pastry overnight in the refrigerator.

4. When ready to prepare pie crust, place one portion of pie pastry and egg white in a large bowl. Using an electric mixer, blend until a soft dough forms.

5. Lightly dust a sheet of parchment paper with rice flour. Form dough into a ball, then flatten into a disk. Place on dusted parchment paper and cover with another sheet of parchment. Using a rolling pin, roll out dough to an 11-inch (28 cm) circle, keeping dough dusted to prevent sticking, flipping dough and paper over to dust both sides. Use as directed in pie recipes.

Hazelnut Pie Pastry

This is a great alternative to the Pie Pastry on page 250 and works especially well for pudding pies or cheesecakes.

Tips

To fit pastry into a pie plate, remove the top sheet of parchment paper and place the pie plate upside down on the pastry. Place your hand under the bottom sheet of parchment and flip the pastry over, easing it into the pie plate. Remove the parchment paper.

If your recipe instructs you to bake the pie pastry before filling it, prick the bottom and sides with a fork. Bake in a 325°F (160°C) oven for 10 to 15 minutes or until edges are golden. Let cool completely before filling.

Nutrients Per 1/6 pie	
Calories	150
Carbohydrate	14 g
Fiber	2 g
Protein	3 g
Fat	10 g
Iron	1 mg
Calcium	12 mg

3/4 cup	freshly ground hazelnuts	175 mL
1/2 cup	sorghum flour	125 mL
2 tbsp	granulated raw cane sugar	30 mL
1/4 tsp	salt	1 mL
2 tbsp	butter, softened	30 mL

1. In a large bowl, combine hazelnuts, flour, sugar and salt. Using a pastry blender or two knives, cut in butter until crumbly. Stir in 1/4 cup (60 mL) water until well combined.

2. When ready to prepare pie crust, lightly dust a sheet of parchment paper with rice flour. Form pastry into a ball, then flatten into a disk. Place on dusted parchment paper and cover with another sheet of parchment. Using a rolling pin, roll out dough to an 11-inch (28 cm) circle, keeping dough dusted with flour. Use as directed in pie recipes.

Pumpkin Pie

This is Theresa's son Eli's favorite pie. She bakes it all year long, as her family can never wait for Thanksgiving.

Tips

If you have a larger can of pumpkin, use 1⅔ cups (400 mL) for this recipe.

Choose your favorite GF non-dairy milk, such as soy, rice, almond or potato-based milk or, if you tolerate lactose, use regular 1% milk.

- Preheat oven to 425°F (220°C)
- 9-inch (23 cm) glass pie plate, greased

	Pie Pastry for one 9-inch (23 cm) single-crust pie (page 250)	
2	eggs, lightly beaten	2
1	can (14 oz/398 mL) pumpkin purée (not pie filling)	1
½ cup	granulated raw cane sugar	125 mL
1 tsp	ground allspice	5 mL
½ tsp	ground cinnamon	2 mL
¼ tsp	salt	1 mL
½ cup	fortified GF non-dairy milk or lactose-free 1% milk	125 mL
1 tsp	vanilla extract	5 mL

1. Fit pastry into pie plate. Set aside.

2. In a large bowl, combine eggs, pumpkin, sugar, allspice, cinnamon, salt, milk and vanilla. Pour into pie shell.

3. Bake in preheated oven for 15 minutes. Reduce heat to 350°F (180°C) and bake for 30 to 40 minutes or until filling is set. Let cool on a wire rack for at least 30 minutes before serving.

Nutrients Per Serving

Calories	190
Carbohydrate	31 g
Fiber	3 g
Protein	5 g
Fat	6 g
Iron	1 mg
Calcium	40 mg

Blueberry and Raspberry Crumble

This yummy crumble can be used to top any combination of fruits you like. Try strawberries and rhubarb, peaches and blueberries, or apples and pears.

Tip

You can use frozen blueberries and raspberries; just increase the baking time by 10 minutes.

- Preheat oven to 350°F (180°C)
- 10- by 7-inch (25 by 18 cm) casserole dish, lightly greased

½ cup	granulated raw cane sugar	125 mL
¼ cup	white rice flour	60 mL
¼ cup	sorghum flour	60 mL
½ tsp	ground cinnamon	2 mL
⅓ cup	cold butter, cut into pieces	75 mL
2 cups	blueberries	500 mL
2 cups	raspberries	500 mL

1. In a large bowl, combine sugar, rice flour, sorghum flour and cinnamon. Using a pastry blender or two knives, cut in butter until mixture resembles coarse crumbs.

2. Place berries in prepared baking dish and sprinkle evenly with crumble.

3. Bake in preheated oven for 20 minutes or until crumble is browned and berries are bubbling.

Nutrients Per Serving	
Calories	340
Carbohydrate	52 g
Fiber	6 g
Protein	3 g
Fat	16 g
Iron	1 mg
Calcium	15 mg

Maple Walnut Tarts

**Makes 12 tarts
(1 per serving)**

Pure maple syrup simply can't be beat. For the best flavor, make sure to use the real thing in these tarts. The combination of maple and walnuts is a classic!

- Preheat oven to 425°F (220°C)
- 3-inch (7.5 cm) round cookie cutter
- 12 paper muffin pan liners
- 12-cup muffin pan

	Pie Pastry for one 9-inch (23 cm) single-crust pie (page 250)	
¼ cup	chopped walnuts	60 mL

Filling

1	egg	1
⅓ cup	pure maple syrup	75 mL
2 tsp	melted butter	10 mL
½ tsp	vanilla extract	2 mL
½ cup	chopped walnuts	125 mL

1. Place pastry on a work surface and roll out to a circle about 12 inches (30 cm) in diameter. Using the cookie cutter, cut out 12 rounds, rerolling scraps if necessary. Spread out one paper liner to a flat circle and place one pastry round in the center. Carefully place into muffin cup. Repeat with remaining paper liners and pastry rounds. Add 1 tsp (5 mL) walnuts to each cup.

2. *Filling:* In a bowl, whisk egg until frothy. Whisk in maple syrup, butter and vanilla until well combined. Stir in walnuts. Pour into prepared muffin cups, dividing evenly.

3. Bake in preheated oven for 12 to 15 minutes or until puffed and golden. Let cool completely in pans on a wire rack.

Nutrients Per Serving	
Calories	150
Carbohydrate	16 g
Fiber	1 g
Protein	3 g
Fat	9 g
Iron	1 mg
Calcium	16 mg

Cake of Goodness

This cake is a breeze to mix up and bake, but the result is so delicious that Theresa's sons and their friends dubbed it Cake of Goodness.

Tip

Choose your favorite GF non-dairy milk, such as soy, rice, almond or potato-based milk or, if you tolerate lactose, use regular 1% milk.

Vegan hard margarine, such as Earth Balance vegan buttery flavor sticks, has almost half as much saturated fat as regular butter and no cholesterol. Where butter is called for in a baking recipe, vegan hard margarine can be a heart-healthy, delicious alternative.

Nutrients Per Serving	
Calories	180
Carbohydrate	30 g
Fiber	1 g
Protein	2 g
Fat	5 g
Iron	0.5 mg
Calcium	48 mg

- Preheat oven to 350°F (180°C)
- 8-inch (20 cm) round metal cake pan, greased, bottom lined with parchment paper

1 cup	white rice flour	250 mL
¾ cup	granulated raw cane sugar	175 mL
½ cup	sorghum flour	125 mL
¼ tsp	salt	1 mL
¼ cup	cold vegan hard margarine or butter, cut into pieces	60 mL
2 tsp	baking powder	10 mL
1 tsp	ground cinnamon	5 mL
1 cup	fortified GF non-dairy milk or lactose-free 1% milk	250 mL
½ tsp	vanilla extract	2 mL
½ tsp	freshly squeezed lemon juice	2 mL

1. In a large bowl, combine rice flour, sugar, sorghum flour and salt. Using a pastry blender or two knives, cut in margarine until mixture resembles coarse crumbs. Reserve ½ cup (125 mL) for topping.

2. To the remaining flour mixture, add baking powder, cinnamon, milk, vanilla and lemon juice; stir until just combined. Pour into prepared baking dish and sprinkle evenly with the reserved flour mixture.

3. Bake in preheated oven for 30 minutes or until a tester inserted in the center comes out clean. Let cool completely in pan on a wire rack.

Easy Peasy Cupcakes

If you have a sweet tooth, you'll love these cupcakes, especially when they're topped with gluten-free icing — though they're good without it, too, if you'd rather do without the extra calories and fat.

Tip

Choose your favorite GF non-dairy milk, such as soy, rice, almond or potato-based milk or, if you tolerate lactose, use regular 1% milk.

Vegan hard margarine, such as Earth Balance vegan buttery flavor sticks, has almost half as much saturated fat as regular butter and no cholesterol. Where butter is called for in a baking recipe, vegan hard margarine can be a heart-healthy, delicious alternative.

- Preheat oven to 350°F (180°C)
- 12-cup muffin pan, greased or lined with paper liners

1 cup	white rice flour	250 mL
2 tsp	GF baking powder	10 mL
¼ tsp	salt	1 mL
½ cup	granulated raw cane sugar	125 mL
⅓ cup	vegan hard margarine or butter, softened	75 mL
1	egg	1
½ tsp	vanilla extract	2 mL
¾ cup	fortified GF non-dairy milk or lactose-free 1% milk	175 mL

1. In a medium bowl, whisk together white rice flour, baking powder and salt.

2. In a large bowl, using an electric mixer, cream sugar and margarine until light and fluffy. Beat in egg, then vanilla, until well combined. Beat in milk until blended. Stir in flour mixture until combined.

3. Spoon batter into prepared muffin cups, dividing equally. Bake in preheated oven for 20 minutes or until golden and a tester inserted in the center comes out clean. Let cool in pan on a wire rack for 5 minutes, then transfer to the rack to cool. These are best served the day they are baked.

Nutrients Per Serving

Calories	120
Carbohydrate	17 g
Fiber	0 g
Protein	2 g
Fat	6 g
Iron	0.2 mg
Calcium	31 mg

This icing is perfect for
Easy Peasy Cupcakes, but
we're sure you'll dream up
other uses for it too!

Easy Peasy Icing

1 cup	instant-dissolving (fruit or berry) sugar	250 mL
½ cup	butter, slightly softened, cut into cubes	125 mL
3 tbsp	unsweetened cocoa powder	45 mL
2 tsp	vanilla extract	10 mL

1. In a bowl, using an electric mixer, cream sugar and butter until fluffy. Beat in cocoa, vanilla and 1 tbsp (15 mL) water for 2 to 3 minutes or until smooth.

Nutrients Per Serving	
Calories	110
Carbohydrate	11 g
Fiber	0 g
Protein	0 g
Fat	8 g
Iron	0.2 mg
Calcium	4 mg

Thanksgiving Cake

In Theresa's home,
Thanksgiving dinner
wouldn't be complete
without this delicious
two-layer spice cake with
a luscious cream cheese
icing spread in the middle
and on the top and sides.
It's an excellent way
to say "Thank you for
everything."

Tip

Vegan hard margarine,
such as Earth Balance
vegan buttery flavor sticks,
has almost half as much
saturated fat as regular
butter and no cholesterol.
Where butter is called for
in a baking recipe, vegan
hard margarine can be a
heart-healthy, delicious
alternative.

Nutrients Per Serving

Calories	360
Carbohydrate	43 g
Fiber	1 g
Protein	6 g
Fat	19 g
Iron	2 mg
Calcium	100 mg

- Preheat oven to 350°F (180°C)
- Two 8-inch (20 cm) round metal cake pans, lightly greased, bottoms lined with parchment paper

¾ cup	sorghum flour	175 mL
¾ cup	brown rice flour	175 mL
2½ tsp	GF baking powder	12 mL
1 tsp	ground cinnamon	5 mL
½ tsp	ground ginger	2 mL
½ tsp	ground nutmeg	2 mL
½ tsp	ground allspice	2 mL
¼ tsp	salt	1 mL
½ cup	granulated raw cane sugar	125 mL
½ cup	vegan hard margarine or butter, softened	125 mL
3	eggs	3
¾ cup	fortified non-dairy GF milk or lactose-free 1% milk	175 mL
⅓ cup	light (fancy) molasses	75 mL

Icing

8 oz	cream cheese, softened	250 g
½ cup	instant-dissolving (fruit or berry) sugar	125 mL
½ tsp	vanilla extract	2 mL

1. In a medium bowl, whisk together sorghum flour, brown rice flour, baking powder, cinnamon, ginger, nutmeg, allspice and salt.

2. In a large bowl, using an electric mixer, cream sugar and margarine until light and fluffy. Beat in eggs, one at a time, until well blended. Beat in milk and molasses until combined. Stir in flour mixture until combined. Pour batter into prepared cake pans, dividing evenly.

3. Bake in preheated oven for 20 to 25 minutes or until a tester inserted in the center comes out clean. Let cool in pans on a wire rack for 5 minutes. Run a knife around the edges of the pans, then invert cakes onto rack. Peel off paper and let cool completely.

Choose your favorite
GF non-dairy milk, such
as soy, rice, almond or
potato-based milk or, if
you tolerate lactose, use
regular 1% milk.

4. *Icing:* In a bowl, using an electric mixer, beat cream cheese, sugar and vanilla until light and fluffy.

5. Place one cake, bottom side up, on a cake plate. Spread top and sides evenly with half the icing. Place second cake, bottom side down, on top. Spread top and sides evenly with the remaining icing. Refrigerate until ready to serve, for up to 1 day.

Pear Sauce

**Makes 6 to
8 servings**

In the fall, when fresh pears
are abundant, try making
this tasty sauce, which
makes a nice alternative
to applesauce when you're
in the mood for a light
dessert.

8	ripe pears, peeled and chopped	8
2 tbsp	water	30 mL
1/2 tsp	ground cinnamon	2 mL
	Whole hazelnuts (optional)	

1. In a medium saucepan, combine pears, water and cinnamon. Bring to a boil over medium-high heat. Cover, reduce heat and simmer, stirring occasionally, for 20 to 30 minutes or until pears are soft.

2. Using a potato masher, mash pears until smooth. Serve sprinkled with hazelnuts, if desired.

Nutrients Per Serving

Calories	100
Carbohydrate	26 g
Fiber	6 g
Protein	1 g
Fat	0 g
Iron	0 mg
Calcium	21 mg

Chocolate Pudding

No one will guess that this chocolatey instant pudding is made with tofu. It's fabulous just as it is or made into a pie (see variation, below).

Variation

Chocolate Pudding Pie:
Prepare Hazelnut Pie Pastry (page 251), fit pastry into a 9-inch (23 cm) glass pie plate, prick the bottom and sides with a fork and bake in a 325°F (160°C) oven for 10 to 15 minutes or until golden. Let cool completely. Prepare a double batch of Chocolate Pudding as instructed at right, but reduce the water to ¼ cup (60 mL). Spread in cooled crust. Refrigerate until chilled.

• Blender

6 oz	drained extra-firm tofu	175 g
½ cup	water	125 mL
½ cup	granulated raw cane sugar	125 mL
¼ cup	unsweetened cocoa powder	60 mL
1 tsp	vanilla extract	5 mL

1. In blender, combine tofu and water; blend until smooth. Add sugar, cocoa and vanilla; blend until well combined, stopping the blender periodically to scrape down pudding from the sides.

2. Transfer to a bowl and serve right away or cover and refrigerate until chilled.

Nutrients Per Serving

Calories	150
Carbohydrate	28 g
Fiber	2 g
Protein	1 g
Fat	5 g
Iron	1 mg
Calcium	40 mg

About the Nutrient Analysis

The nutrient analysis done on the recipes in this book was derived from the Food Processor Nutrition Analysis Software, version 10.5.0, ESHA Research (2009).

Where necessary, data was supplemented using the following references:

1. Shelley Case, Gluten-Free Diet: A Comprehensive Resource Guide, Expanded Edition (Regina, SK: Case Nutrition Consulting, 2006).

2. Bob's Red Mill Natural Foods. Nutritional information product search. Retrieved April 15, 2009, from www.bobsredmill. com/catalog/index.php?action=search.

3. Gluten-free oats and oat flour from Cream Hill Estates (www. creamhillestates.com). Certificate of Analysis of Pure Oats (Lasalle, QC: Silliker Canada Co., 2005). Certificate of Analysis of Oat Flour (Lasalle, QC: Silliker Canada Co., 2006).

4. Mary's Gone Crackers. Nutritional information product search. Retrieved November 10, 2009, from www. marysgonecrackers.com/product_info. php?products_id=1.

5. Agropur Inc. Natrel 1% MF lactose-free milk nutritional information product search. Retrieved July 1, 2010, from www.natrel.ca/nutrition_shared/nut_ natrel_lactose_1.html.

6. Earth Balance Natural Spreads. Vegan Buttery Sticks nutritional information product search. Retrieved September 28, 2009, from www.earthbalancenatural. com/eb_pdfs/products/vegan-sticks- nutrition-info.pdf.

7. Earth Balance Natural Spreads. Vegan Natural Shortening nutritional information product search. Retrieved December 5, 2009, from www. earthbalancenatural.com/eb_pdfs/ products/shortening-nutrition-info.pdf.

8. Rizopia. Spiral Brown Rice Pasta nutritional information product search. Package Nutrition Facts. Retrieved December 16, 2009, from www.rizopia. com/M1Sel2.htm.

9. Food Directions Inc. Tinkyáda Lasagne with Rice Bran nutritional information product search. Package Nutrition Facts. Retrieved November 11, 2009.

10. Unico Foods Canada. Marinated Artichoke Hearts in Oil nutritional information product search. Retrieved July 17, 2010, from http://www.unico.ca/ cgi-bin/products.cgi.

11. Unico Foods Canada. Romano Beans nutritional information product search. Retrieved July 17, 2010, from http:// www.unico.ca/cgi-bin/products.cgi.

Recipes were evaluated as follows:

- The larger number of servings was used where there is a range.
- Where alternatives are given, the first ingredient and amount listed were used.
- Optional ingredients and ingredients that are not quantified were not included.
- Calculations were based on imperial measures and weights.
- Nutrient values were rounded to the nearest whole number.
- Calculations involving meat and poultry used lean portions without skin.
- Canola oil was used where the type of fat was not specified.
- Recipes were analyzed prior to cooking.

It is important to note that the cooking method used to prepare the recipe may alter the nutrient content per serving, as may ingredient substitutions and differences among brand-name products.

Library and Archives Canada Cataloguing in Publication

Anca, Alexandra
    Complete gluten-free diet & nutrition guide : with a 30 day meal plan &
over 100 recipes / Alexandra Anca ; with Theresa Santandrea-Cull

Includes index.
ISBN 978-0-7788-0252-5

    1. Gluten-free diet. 2. Gluten-free diet--Recipes. 3. Celiac disease--Diet therapy.
I. Santandrea-Cull, Theresa, 1958- II. Title. III. Title: Complete gluten-free diet
and nutrition guide.

RM237.86.A54 2010   641.5'638   C2010-903262-4

Index